THE GREAT PHYSICIAN'S

R^x *for*

DEPRESSION AND ANXIETY

JORDAN RUBIN

with *Joseph Brasco, M.D.*

THOMAS NELSON
Since 1798

NASHVILLE   DALLAS   MEXICO CITY   RIO DE JANEIRO   BEIJING

Every effort has been made to make this book as accurate as possible. The purpose of this book is to educate. It is a review of scientific evidence that is presented for information purposes. No individual should use the information in this book for self-diagnosis, treatment, or justification in accepting or declining any medical therapy for any health problems or diseases. No individual is discouraged from seeking professional medical advice and treatment, and this book is not supplying medical advice.

Any application of the information herein is at the reader's own discretion and risk. Therefore, any individual with a specific health problem or who is taking medications must first seek advice from his personal physician or health-care provider before starting a health and wellness program. The author and Thomas Nelson Publishers, Inc., shall have neither liability nor responsibility to any person or entity with respect to loss, damage, or injury caused or alleged to be caused directly or indirectly by the information contained in this book. We assume no responsibility for errors, inaccuracies, omissions, or any inconsistency herein.

In view of the complex, individual nature of health problems, this book and the ideas, programs, procedures, and suggestions herein are not intended to replace the advice of trained medical professionals. All matters regarding one's health require medical supervision. A physician should be consulted prior to adopting any program or programs described in this book. The author and publisher disclaim any liability arising directly or indirectly from the use of this book.

Copyright © 2007 by Jordan Rubin

Published in Nashville, Tennessee. Thomas Nelson is a trademark of Thomas Nelson, Inc.

Thomas Nelson Inc. titles may be purchased in bulk for educational, business, fundraising, or sales promotional use. For information, please e-mail SpecialMarkets@ThomasNelson.com.

All Scripture quotations, unless otherwise indicated, are taken from The New King James Version (NKJV), Copyright © 1979, 1980, 1982, Thomas Nelson, Inc., Publishers.

Other Scripture references are from the following sources:

The Holy Bible, New International Version (NIV). Copyright © 1973, 1978, 1984. International Bible Society. Used by permission of Zondervan Bible Publishers.

The King James Version of the Bible (KJV).

Library of Congress Cataloging-in-Publication Data

Rubin, Jordan.
    The great physician's RX for depression and anxiety / Jordan Rubin, with Joseph Brasco.
      p. cm.
    ISBN 978-0-7852-1920-0
    1. Depression, Mental—Prevention—Popular works. 2. Anxiety—Prevention—Popular works. 3. Depression, Mental—Religious aspects—Christianity. 4. Anxiety—Religious aspects—Christianity. I. Brasco, Joseph. II. Title.
RC537.R83 2007
616.85'27061—dc22   2007014388

Printed in the United States of America

07 08 09 10 11 QW 5 4 3 2 1

CONTENTS

INTRODUCTION

Down for the Count

I met Ryan Feasel after speaking at a church in northwest Ohio, and his startling story sounded like something out of *A Beautiful Mind*, the 2001 movie starring Russell Crowe as John Nash, the brilliant but asocial mathematician whose life took a nightmarish turn after he accepted secret work in cryptography during the height of the Cold War. The riveting film won the Oscar for Best Picture the following year.

Like John Nash, Ryan was a math teacher—a junior high math and science teacher in Dayton, Ohio, and Indianapolis, Indiana. His problems started at eight years of age when his six-year-old sister, Tricia, died after suffering for years from lupus. The event profoundly saddened Ryan, and his young mind constantly wondered if he could have done something that could have saved the life of his only sibling.

A few years later, he began acting out obsessive-compulsive behavior. Once when he was in elementary school, Ryan was washing dishes for his mom. He looked up and saw dust filtering through sunlight outside the kitchen window. Because he was convinced that dust was dirtying his clean dishes, Ryan washed every single plate and glass over again.

As this type of behavior followed him into adulthood, Ryan's weight ballooned to 350 pounds, resulting in severe digestive issues, blood sugar problems, and heart palpitations. But even worse, he couldn't turn off his mind. It was always sending intrusive thoughts and images into his head, where they would lodge themselves and rule his life. "I couldn't be rational," he said. "That's why obsessive-compulsive disorder is called the 'doubting disease.'"

For instance, Ryan once read Mark 3:28–30, which says "Assuredly, I say to you, all sins will be forgiven the sons of men, and whatever blasphemies they may utter; but he who blasphemes against the Holy Spirit never has forgiveness, but is subject to eternal condemnation" (NKJV).

Ryan doubted himself. He really wasn't sure if he had committed the "unpardonable sin." The more he obsessed about it, the more he worried that he had inadvertently blasphemed the Holy Spirit, which meant he was doomed. For the next six months, Ryan called every pastor in his county asking for clarification, worried that he was going straight to hell. That's when Ryan sought professional help and learned, at the age of nineteen, that he had moderate to severe obsessive-compulsive disorder and severe clinical depression. A psychiatrist put him on a heavy load of antidepressant medicines.

Ryan soldiered on and earned a teaching degree, but once in the classroom, his churning mind wondered what it would be like to make offhand negative or weird comments to his impressionable junior high students. Not that he wanted to, but . . .

Wracked by remorse, Ryan felt so guilty about this possibility that he banged his head against the doorway leading into his classroom, causing a concussion. Eventually, the young teacher couldn't handle being in the classroom, so he applied for disability, which was approved. Out of a teaching job, he moved back in with his parents.

"My obsessive-compulsive disorder has made my life unbearable at times," he said. "Like so many sufferers, I'm often very embarrassed of the things I found my brain telling me I should do. I've done my best to hide this from others."

One night Ryan was surfing the Internet, desperate to help his mental condition as well as his physical health. He was sure he would die prematurely because of his morbidly obese weight. Then he found me, and my books, on the Internet. After learning about the Great Physician's prescription, Ryan radically changed his diet to organic foods and dumped the processed junk in the trash. He ate a lot of buffalo and other grass-fed meat. He ate free-range omega-3 eggs with bright orange yolks.

Besides eating much healthier, Ryan began taking nutritional supplements like probiotics with soil-based organisms (SBOs) and digestive enzymes, as well as omega-3 cod liver oil, which helped a great deal. He also began exercising and lifting weights at the local YMCA, but again, it was one step forward, two steps backward at times. He became obsessed about his weight-lifting technique.

"I could be bench-pressing 120 pounds, and I could take two or three hours to finish my reps," he said. "That's because I was obsessed with my hand position, arch of my back, and my extension—anything the mind forced me to figure a way to correct. I would feel more comfortable walking in downtown Baghdad than having to deal with the pain and torture I endured in my mind each day. If those reading this have obsessive-compulsive behavior, depression, and crippling anxiety, then they'll know what I'm talking about, but there is hope. I don't know where I'd be today without the Great Physician's prescription."

I was greatly impressed when I met Ryan, who is now thirty-six years old. Although he's still on disability, he's jogging on the comeback road. Since following the plan outlined in *The Great Physician's Rx for Depression and Anxiety*, he's lost 140 pounds. He now weighs a solid 210 pounds, thanks to those fervent weight-training sessions in the gym. I'm looking forward to seeing where his future goes.

I feel for folks like Ryan, who are battling a variety of depression and anxiety disorders, from obsessive-compulsive behaviors like a hand-washing Howard Hughes to dealing with major bouts of the blues. On a personal note, I had my own battle with depression when I faced a life-threatening illness at nineteen years of age. (I'll describe that situation in greater detail in Key #7: "Live a Life of Prayer and Purpose.")

In addition, depression certainly played a role when my mother's first cousin took her own life, as well as one of Mom's best friends. One of my sister's best friends committed suicide. A former employee who was severely depressed with postpartum depression drowned her infant son, and believe it or not, a second former employee murdered her husband and took her own life. (Both of the aforementioned events took place a few years after these employees left my organization.)

The point here is that depression and anxiety have become extremely common. Thus, I don't take depression and anxiety lightly, and I'm sure you don't either. The ranks of the depressed are increasing all the time, and according to the latest US government statistics, around nineteen million Americans suffer from clinical depression, according to the National Institutes of Health (NIH).[1] Symptoms may include:

- overwhelming feelings of panic and fear
- uncontrollable obsessive thoughts
- painful, intrusive memories
- recurring nightmares
- physical symptoms, such as feeling sick to your stomach, heart pounding, and muscle tension

Ryan Feasel could place a checkmark next to each symptom, and perhaps you or someone you love can do so as well. Depression and anxiety affect your thoughts, your moods, your feelings, your behavior, your sleep, your eating habits, your career, your sex life, and your relationships with family and friends. Episodes of depression can range from mild to severe, and they can happen as a single occurrence or as recurring episodes. If depression symptoms last more than two years, then the disorder is characterized as "chronic." When someone's mood cycles between depression and mania, he or she is said to have manic depression or bipolar disorder.

Left untreated, depression can set off a downward spiral that leads to disability, dependency, and even suicide.

A Depressing State

Depression may be a coping mechanism for the body, a sign that responsibilities or situations beyond our control are overwhelming, says the *Encyclopedia of Natural Healing*. A precipitous or life-changing event, such as the death of a loved one, a business reversal, or a busted relationship can trigger an emotional trauma that leads to recurring bouts of depression. Even a streak of dark, gloomy weather in the dead of winter can give people a dose of the blues.

Anxiety, on the other hand, represents a state of emotional turmoil characterized by fearfulness and apprehension. Either way, depression and anxiety are equal-opportunity mental health conditions and global in scope. They affect people of all ages, races, and nationalities, but the World Health Organization (WHO) calls depression the most costly of all diseases because of the way it disables people who would otherwise be productive.

Women are twice as likely as men to develop depression.[2] According to the National Institutes of Health, clinical depression will affect up to 25 percent of women in their lifetimes and up to 12 percent of men. Adolescents are easily susceptible to feeling depressed, as witnessed by today's teen suicide rates.

Depression and anxiety alter the chemistry of your body, which can be a pervasive force in determining your daily behavior. Apathy and helplessness cause a cycle of passivity and helplessness, which further erodes self-confidence. Women, more so than men, seem to beat themselves up emotionally for doing something stupid, saying the wrong thing, or allowing themselves to gain far more weight than they ever thought possible. Whether you're male or female, not dealing with emotional issues leads to stress, anger, self-pity, and resentment.

If you're having difficulty enjoying life or doing things that were once pleasurable, you're said to be depressed if you've experienced at least five of the following symptoms for the last two weeks or more:

1. Sleep disturbances (at least 90 percent of people with depression have either insomnia [sleeplessness] or hypersomnia [excessive sleeping]).

2. Significant change in appetite, often resulting in weight loss or weight gain.

3. Fatigue or loss of energy.

4. Feelings of worthlessness, self-hate, and inappropriate guilt.

5. Extreme difficulty concentrating.

6. Either agitation, restlessness, irritability, inactivity, or withdrawal.

7. Recurring thoughts of death or suicide.

8. Feelings of hopelessness.[3]

As this list demonstrates, you can't link depression to a single cause, although scientists believe an imbalance in brain chemicals—called neurotransmitters—results in depression. Scientists don't understand how imbalances in these neurotransmitters, which are known as serotonin, norepinephrine, and dopamine, cause fatigue or feelings of hopelessness, but they do. Here are other factors that contribute to depression:

Heredity. Family ties play a big role in who becomes depressed. Up to 50 percent of people suffering from depression had one or two parents who displayed similar symptoms of feeling worthless, hopeless, guilty, irritable, or angry, according to *Prescription for Nutritional Healing*.[4] A study in the *American Journal of Psychiatry* showed that chronic depression can strike more than once in an immediate family. Researchers also found that relatives were six times more likely to have chronic depression if their family member had become chronically depressed by age thirteen.[5]

Stress. Losing a job, a business reversal, or looming bankruptcy creates unwanted stress.

Illnesses. Learning that you have a serious, life-threatening disease, such as cancer, diabetes, Alzheimer's, or a heart condition, puts you at a higher risk of developing depression.

Personality. If you're eternally pessimistic, the type who always sees the glass half-empty, you're vulnerable to depression.

Alcohol and drug use. Steady drinking and hallucinogenic drugs throw you into life's pit, where you feel even more worthless— and depressed. Smoking is another vice that doesn't leave one happier.

Hormones. Guys may joke that PMS stands for "permissible man slaughter," but women know that when their hormones swirl on the eve of their menstrual cycle, they're candidates for mood swings, bloating, and irritability. Around 10 percent of menstruating women experience PMS symptoms so severe that it causes outbursts of anger, even suicidal thoughts, while interfering with job performance and family relationships.[6]

Postpartum Blues

There's no doubt that childbirth is an emotionally intense event, but I found out how much so after my wife, Nicki, and I brought our firstborn child, Joshua, home from the hospital three years ago. For the first couple of weeks, Nicki experienced a minor case of the "baby blues," which doctors say is a fairly common experience for 80 percent of new moms. Doctors characterize "baby blues" as crying spells, mood swings, and irritability beginning three days after birth.

Women who don't get over the baby blues after a couple of weeks, however, may develop postpartum depression, which happens to more than 10 percent of new moms.[7] They may experience a sense of being overwhelmed, an inability to sleep, or poor appetite.

Doctors say postpartum depression is caused by hormonal shifts that happen after childbirth, when a woman's levels of estrogen and progesterone rapidly fall to nonpregnant levels. The change in hormone levels prompts reactions sleeplessness including crabbiness, mental confusion, and even psychosis. Postpartum depression is very real, which is why it's critical for young mothers to cry out for help, seek counseling, and talk with their doctors.

As for Nicki, she mitigated the "baby blues" by eating as well as she could before and after Joshua's birth, taking supplements, practicing advanced hygiene so she wouldn't get sick, and remaining as active as her body would allow—keys that are part of the Great Physician's prescription.

Why are so many people walking the face of this earth feeling depressed and anxious about the present or the future? Why are so many Christians depressed as well? Judging from the numbers of depressed people who meet with me after I speak at churches and conferences, I would say that too many of us in the Church are hurting from depression and anxiety. Yet Scripture is full of reminders from God not to stress out over everyday life:

- "Therefore do not worry . . . But seek first the kingdom of God and His righteousness, and all these things shall be added to you" (Matt. 6:31, 33 NKJV).

- "Are not two sparrows sold for a copper coin? And not one of them falls to the ground apart from your Father's will. But the very hairs of your head are all numbered. Do not fear therefore; you are of more value than many sparrows" (Matt. 10:29–31 NKJV).

- "Be anxious for nothing, but in everything by prayer and supplication, with thanksgiving, let your requests be made known to God; and the peace of God, which surpasses all understanding, will guard your hearts and minds through Christ Jesus" (Phil. 4:6–7 NKJV).

- "Then He spoke a parable to them, that men always ought to pray and not lose heart" (Luke 18:1 NKJV).

And finally, one of the all-time best verses in the Bible:

- "Come to Me, all you who labor and are heavy laden, and I will give you rest. Take My yoke upon you and learn from Me, for I am gentle and lowly in heart, and you will find rest for your souls. For My yoke is easy and My burden is light" (Matt. 11:28–30 NKJV).

The yoke around our necks these days are our complicated, hyper-speed, shop-until-we-drop, always-on-the-go lives. At a recent medical conference, Julia Ross, the best-selling author of *The Mood Cure*, said that when you take the population as a whole, we're one hundred times more depressed today than folks were one hundred years ago.[8] Just in the last twelve years, adult depression and anxiety levels have tripled.[9] Ms. Ross added that panic attacks are the biggest reason why heart disease is climbing among women.

Why so many depressed people today? After all, adults have always been subjected to various levels of stress over the centuries: waiting for rain to fall on crops, lack of medical care, twelve-hour workdays, no clean water, and nothing to eat. But life—at least from our modern-day perspective—certainly looks revved up and terribly complicated today just because of the *speed* at which we live. We don't cope well with 24/7 lifestyles, but I can't help but wonder how big a role nutritional deficiencies, a lack of exercise, and no time to "smell the roses," among other things, is playing with modern-day depression and anxiety.

CONVENTIONAL TREATMENT

Researchers at the University of Washington had a pretty good idea a few years ago: What would happen if we sent actors pretending to be patients into doctor's offices and have them complain about symptoms of stress and fatigue? Would they exit with a prescription for an antidepressant medication?

That's exactly what University of Washington researchers did when they dispatched actors to 152 doctors' offices. Not only did those who faked symptoms of depression receive prescriptions, but more than half of those (55 percent) who did *not* report any symptoms were written a prescription for the antidepressant drug Paxil when they asked for it by name, underscoring how compliant doctors were to go along with their patients' requests.[10] Now you know why those bright and cheery TV ads remind you to "ask your doctor about Paxil" or whatever drug they are promoting.

I'm afraid that too many physicians, when facing a patient complaining about feeling depressed, reach for their prescription pads to solve the problem. Conventional medicine's approach to treatment for depression can be summed up from this statement from the Mayo Clinic Web site: "Medication can relieve symptoms of depression and have become the first line of treatment for this disorder."[11]

There's some big money behind the push for antidepressant drugs. Big Pharma, as the medical press calls the world's prescription drug makers, sold an estimated ten billion dollars' worth of antidepressants in 2005, the year with the most recent data.[12] Brand names like Zoloft, Lexapro, Paxil, Wellbutrin, and Prozac take a lion's share of that business. Zoloft is the top-selling antidepressant and sixth mostpopular drug overall, racking up retail sales of more than $2.5 billion.[13] (Pfizer, the maker of Zoloft, lost its patent in 2006, making it available to makers of generic drugs.)

What's amazing to me is the number of prescriptions written for antidepressants in a year. Want to guess how many? The Top twenty psychiatric prescriptions dispensed in 2005, from Xanax to Paxil, added up to *256 million* prescriptions. That's a lot of refills![14]

There are several classes of antidepressants, but the most popular are selective serotonin reuptake inhibitors, or SSRIs. This class of drug increases—or rather sustains—the activity of serotonin, a neurotransmitter in the brain. SSRIs, as you would expect for potent drugs these days, come with a host of side effects: upset stomach, weight gain, drowsiness, sexual dysfunction (such as impotence, decreased libido, and diminished orgasm), headaches, and apathy.

If the new mood-stabilizing drugs fail to improve the patient's depression, a physician may suggest psychotherapy, which can help one cope with any problems in his or her life that would be causing feelings of depression.

Chasing away the demons of depression and anxiety isn't easy. Some people respond well to antidepressants and feel like they are getting back on track. For others, depression camps out at their doorstep and sticks around for a long time. In about 20 to 30 percent of people who have an episode of depression, the symptoms don't go away entirely.[15]

Teens and Antidepressants

The Food and Drug Administration has directed manufacturers of antidepressant drugs to add "black box" warnings that describe the increased risk of suicide in children and adolescents given antidepressant medications.

There's a good reason for the FDA to take this measure: teen suicide. In 2006, GlaxoSmithKline, the makers of the antidepressant drug Paxil, conducted clinical trials on nearly fifteen thousand patients and found a higher frequency of suicidal behavior among the young adults treated with the drug.[16]

ALTERNATIVE TREATMENT

Some people don't want to go through life on antidepressants because of the strength-sapping side effects or the foggy feeling that they're sleepwalking during their waking hours. An increasing number are seeking out alternative therapies—a more "holistic" approach—to deal with their depression and anxiety.

Alternative treatments center around herbal and dietary supplements. The most popular supplement marketed for depression is St. John's wort, an extract of a weedy plant that increases deep sleep and reduces anxiety, says *Psychology Today* magazine. It has been used to treat "nervous disorders" for centuries. The herb may also work like antidepressant drugs in inhibiting the brain's uptake of serotonin and norepinephrine. St. John's wort is so popular in Germany that two hundred thousand prescriptions were written for it several years ago.[17]

Prescription for Natural Cures' top recommendation for depression is taking a natural compound of two molecules called S-adenosyllmethionine, or SAMe. "A double-blind study at the University of California Irvine Medical Center found that 62 percent of people taking SAMe and 52 percent of those taking a pharmaceutical antidepressant improved significantly," according to *Prescription for Natural Cures*.[18]

Another alternative therapy finding favor is acupuncture, which is the Chinese practice of inserting needles into the body at specific points. Practitioners say that acupuncture can help regulate the body's flow of energy as well as emotional changes, which can reduce symptoms of depression.

Researchers from the University of Arizona, John Nlen, Ph.D., and Sabdna Hitt, Ph.D., conducted a study to see if the healing art of acupuncture could alleviate symptoms of depression. Thirty-eight clinically depressed women were divided into three groups, and 50 percent of those who received acupuncture treatments for depression showed no sign of the mood disorder within two months. After the initial testing period, the researchers gave all thirty-eight depressed women acupuncture treatment, after which 70 percent of them experienced a drop in depressive symptoms.[19]

Finally, some people believe in relaxation therapy, which is accomplished through completing structured exercises for relaxing both the body and the mind. The same goes for massage therapy, slow breathing exercises, and periods of stretching, which are reputed to have calming effects on the psyche.

WHERE WE GO FROM HERE

Michael Gershon, M.D., a neurobiologist at New York City's Columbia-Presbyterian Medical Center, has devoted his career to studying the human bowel—the stomach, esophagus, small intestine, and colon. His thirty years of research have led to an electrifying discovery that relates to depression and anxiety: nerve cells in the gut act like another brain in the body.

What happens is that the nervous system in our gut, which contains an independent network of over half of the body's nerve cells, acts like a "second brain," and the entire gastrointestinal system is the body's second nervous system. "The brain is not the only place in the body that's full of neurotransmitters," Dr. Gershon explained. "One hundred million neurotransmitters line the length of the gut—approximately the same number found in the brain."[20]

So, if you've ever had butterflies in your stomach before addressing an audience—or before playing a big game—the "second brain" in your gut is producing emotion-based feelings.

Your two brains communicate back and forth by way of a nerve trunk extending from the base of the brain all the way down to your abdomen. When one brain is upset, the other knows about it right away.

Since neurotransmitters such as serotonin are located in the gut, it affects many critical things in people's lives, suggests Dr. Gershon. "It affects their mood, so that if it's abnormal, they get depressed. It affects how much they eat, it affects how much sex they have, and it affects how the bowel works."[21]

In other words, some depression will manifest as *physical* symptoms: irritable bowel syndrome (IBS), constipation, diarrhea, and Crohn's disease. Another New York doctor, John Sarno, M.D., a professor of clinical rehabilitation medicine at New York University Medical Center, explored the crucial interaction between a rational, conscious mind and the repressed feelings of emotional pain that are the basis for many "mind-body" disorders, as he calls them in his book *The Divided Mind: The Epidemic of Mindbody Disorders*. Dr. Sarno theorized that deadly emotions such as depression and anxiety could stimulate the brain to manufacture physical symptoms like back pain, migraine headaches, and even acne.

This is where the Great Physician's prescription for depression and anxiety comes in. I recommend a total lifestyle program for the health of the body, mind, and spirit that's more comprehensive than a prescription for antidepressants. My plan is based on the 7 Keys to unlock your God-given health potential, discussed in my foundational book *The Great Physician's Rx for Health and Wellness*. They are:

- Key #1: Eat to live.

- Key #2: Supplement your diet with whole food nutritionals, living nutrients, and superfoods.

- Key #3: Practice advanced hygiene.

- Key #4: Condition your body with exercise and body therapies.

- Key #5: Reduce toxins in your environment.

- Key #6: Avoid deadly emotions.

- Key #7: Live a life of prayer and purpose.

These keys are part of a healthy lifestyle that will lift your mood, provide the body with the right fuel to feel energized during the day, and give you a purpose for living. I'm one of those who believes that depression and anxiety require a positive attitude. This is the time to focus on your abilities, not your disabilities. This is the time to rebuild your health, brick by brick. And this is the time to develop daily routines that maximize your quality of life and minimize your dark days.

I'm convinced there's a light at the end of the tunnel. Better health and better attitudes won't happen overnight, but I'm confident the Great Physician's prescription can work for you because I've spoken or received e-mails from plenty of folks describing how the Great Physician's health principles helped them turn their lives around.

I believe each and every one of us has a God-given health

potential that can be unlocked, but only with the right keys. I want to challenge you to incorporate these timeless principles and allow God to transform your health as you leave depression and anxiety behind and look forward to a future with hope.

KEY #1

Eat to Live

If you don't think there's a link between food and mood, then why do people call a home-cooked meal with meat loaf, mashed potatoes, green beans, and apple pie "comfort food"?

Everyone feels his or her mood lift after Mom cooks a well-rounded meal made from scratch and served with love. Now there's scientific evidence showing that how you feel emotionally is greatly affected, good or bad, by what you choose to chew on and swallow. According to a major report from the Mental Health Foundation in the United Kingdom, depression and anxiety could be due to a poor diet that lacks the essential ingredients to keep the brain healthy.[1]

The report, called "Feeding Minds," said that the brain relies on a mixture of complex carbohydrates, essential fatty acids (EFAs) such as omega-3 and omega-6, vitamins, and water to work properly. Nutritional deficiency in any of these areas could seriously hamper the body's ability to make neurotransmitters such as serotonin, one of the major neurotransmitters that affects your mood.

Too many depressed individuals think they can enjoy their favorite dessert and feel better about themselves, but that's not the case. "Seeking solace in a handful of chocolate chip cookies is a quick solution, usually regretted by the time we're swiping the crumbs from our mouth," says registered dietician Elizabeth

1

Somers, author of *Food & Mood: The Complete Guide to Eating Well and Feeling Your Best.*

The fact of the matter is that choices you make on what to eat set the tone for your physical *and* mental health. We know that low serotonin levels result in depression, and serotonin has been called the brain's own mood-elevating drug. We also know that the manufacture of serotonin in the brain depends upon how much tryptophan—an amino acid—reaches that part of the body. It doesn't take Albert Einstein to realize that eating foods high in tryptophan would be a good idea if a doctor handed you a prescription for Zoloft.

What are some foods that provide the brain with this important amino acid? Well, bananas, dates, figs, tuna, whole grains, and especially yogurt and turkey are good examples. Foods *low* in tryptophan would be jelly-filled doughnuts, bacon cheeseburgers, chili fries, candy bars, deep-dish Italian sausage pizza, and chocolate chip ice cream, which pretty much outlines what many Americans eat these days.

If you want to keep your focus sharp, your concentration keen, and your mood up, then eat fresh fruits, whole grains, and fresh fish and meat, which are just some of the natural foods that are part of the Great Physician's prescription first key—"Eat to Live." You take a big step toward beating back depression and anxiety when you do these two things:

1. Eat what God created for food.
2. Eat food in a form that is healthy for the body.

As you will see in this chapter, following these two vital principles will give you a great shot toward living a healthy, vibrant, and upbeat life.

BACK TO THE SOURCE

What are some foods that God created? My friend Rex Russell, M.D., compiled a comprehensive list in his book *What the Bible Says About Healthy Living*. I'm reprinting them here, along with the scriptural references. As you scan through his list, ask yourself if these sound like foods that Moses and the Israelites would have consumed:

- almonds (Gen. 43:11)
- barley (Judg. 7:13)
- beans (Ezek. 4:9)
- bread (1 Sam. 17:17)
- broth (Judg. 6:19)
- cakes, and probably not the kind with frosting (2 Sam. 13:8 NKJV)
- cheese (Job 10:10)
- cucumbers, onions, leeks, melons, and garlic (Num. 11:5)
- curds of cow's milk (Deut. 32:14)
- figs (Num. 13:23)
- fish (Matt. 7:10)

- fowl (1 Kings 4:23)
- fruit (2 Sam. 16:2)
- game (Gen. 25:28)
- goat's milk (Prov. 27:27)
- grain (Ruth 2:14)
- grapes (Deut. 23:24)
- grasshoppers, locusts, and crickets (Lev. 11:22)
- herbs (Exod. 12:8)
- honey (Isa. 7:15) and wild honey (Ps. 19:10)
- lentils (Gen. 25:34)
- meal (Matt. 13:33 KJV)
- pistachio nuts (Gen. 43:11)
- oil (Prov. 21:17)
- olives (Deut. 28:40)
- pomegranates (Num. 13:23)
- quail (Num. 11:32)
- raisins (2 Sam. 16:1)
- salt (Job 6:6)
- sheep (Deut. 14:4)
- sheep's milk (Deut. 32:14)
- spices (Gen. 43:11)
- veal (Gen. 18:7–8)
- vegetables (Prov. 15:17)
- vinegar (Num. 6:3)[2]

Have these foods been staples in your diet? Do you have to think hard to remember the last time you bit into a fresh apple, scooped up a handful of raisins, ate a cup of sheep's milk yogurt, or supped on lentil soup? These listed foods are nutritional gold mines and contain no refined or processed carbohydrates and no artificial sweeteners. Since God has given us a bountiful harvest of natural foods to eat, it would take several pages to describe all the fantastic fruits and vibrant vegetables available from His garden. A diet based on whole and natural foods fits within the bull's-eye of eating foods that God created in a form healthy for the body.

I believe God gave us physiologies that crave these foods in their natural state because our bodies are genetically set for certain nutritional requirements by our Creator. Our taste buds, however, have been manipulated by fast-food chains and restaurants that sweeten meats with secret sauces and top everything in sight with melted cheese and bacon. The strategy has worked: we've become a country that loves inexpensive deep-fried, greasy food. For many of us, taste trumps health, which explains why drive-thru chains and sit-down restaurants are doing great business serving cheese-and-egg sandwiches, monster burgers, pail-sized barrels of fried chicken, and stuffed-crust pizza—foods not in a form that God created.

Having an awareness of what you eat is an important first step to dealing with depression and anxiety. As we begin traveling down this road together, I need to help you understand that everything you eat is a protein, a fat, or a carbohydrate—nutrients needed to sustain ongoing serotonin production in the brain. Each of these nutrients can positively or negatively affect how you feel.

Let's take a closer look at these macronutrients.

The First Word on Protein

Proteins, one of the basic components of foods, are the essential building blocks of the body. All proteins are combinations of twenty-two amino acids, which build body organs, muscles, and nerves, to name a few important duties. Among other things, proteins provide for the transport of nutrients, oxygen, and waste throughout the body and are required for the structure, function, and regulation of the body's cells, tissues, and organs. Protein builds muscle, repairs damaged tissues, and strengthens our immune systems.

Our bodies, however, cannot produce all twenty-two amino acids that we need to live a robust life. Scientists have discovered that eight essential amino acids are missing, meaning that they must come from sources outside the body. Since we need these eight amino acids badly, it just so happens that animal protein—chicken, beef, lamb, dairy, eggs, and so on—is the only complete protein source providing the Big Eight amino acids.

Tryptophan is an essential amino acid, which means that it must be obtained through the diet in adequate quantities. If we don't eat enough foods with tryptophan, the body doesn't have the raw materials it needs to produce the neurotransmitter serotonin. The richest dietary sources of tryptophan include poultry, meat, fish and dairy, as I mentioned earlier.

The best meat comes from organically raised, grass-fed cattle, sheep, goats, buffalo, and venison—animals that graze on pastureland grasses. Grass-fed meat and free-range poultry are leaner and lower in calories than grain-fed meat. But more importantly for those suffering from depression, these healthy meats deliver the best source of tryptophan to your body.

I don't believe that the best and most healthy sources of animal protein come from your supermarket's meat case. Commercially raised livestock and poultry are routinely fed grain and meal laced with hormones, nitrates, and pesticides—chemicals that have been investigated as possible carcinogenic substances. In this country, cattle routinely chew on feedstuffs with hormones (melengestrol acetate, or MGA) and buffers (sodium bicarbonate). These additives help livestock owners fatten up their herd—which fattens their bottom lines—but these practices don't provide you with the most nutritious meat.

The same goes for free-range, pasture-fed poultry, which is the antithesis of modern methods of chicken production. These days, commercially raised chickens are brutally de-beaked, raised in long, windowless sheds, cooped up without fresh air, and fed from hoppers dispensing food pellets and water. Talk about depressing! These chickens live miserable lives until they're plump enough to slaughter, as compared to their country cousins, who are allowed to roam around and hunt and peck for their food.

Here's another reason why you should be eating organic meat instead of commercial cuts. We know that the brain also needs two types of essential fatty acids, (EFAs), omega-3 and omega-6, for the production of neurotransmitters like serotonin. Both of these EFAs are bountiful in leafy plants consumed by roaming animals. The fat in wild game and grass-fed animals contains roughly *seven* times more omega-3 fatty acids than animals raised for commercial meat.[3]

Fish are also well known for being excellent sources of omega-3 and omega-6 essential fatty acids. Salmon and other cold-water fish contain high levels of these beneficial EFAs, which may hold the key to naturally easing depression, as confirmed by this ABC News report:

Studies have shown that in countries where large amounts of fish are consumed, rates of depression are low as compared with countries where little fish is consumed. This has led researchers to examine whether omega-3 fats found in fish are responsible for the decreased evidence of depression . . . and some psychiatrists are now recommending that their depressed patients increase their consumption of these fatty acids."[4]

I think that's a great idea. To take in the best omega-3 essential fatty acids, you should shop for fish with scales and fins caught in the wild from oceans and rivers and not "feedlot salmon" raised on fish farms, which don't compare to their cold-water cousins in terms of taste or nutritional value. The salmon from fish farms spend several years lazily circling concrete tanks, fattening up on pellets of salmon chow, not streaking through the ocean eating small marine life as they're supposed to. While it's great to see more people eating the tender meat of farm-raised Atlantic salmon—albeit colored with orange dye—it's never going to nutritionally match what comes from the wild.

Wild-caught fish is an absolutely incredible food and should be consumed liberally. Look for "Alaskan" or "wild-caught" on the label at your local fish market or health food store. Be aware that you can now find delicious high omega-3, low mercury canned tuna, which has nearly twice the omega-3 fats per serving of wild-caught salmon. (For more information, visit www.BiblicalHealth Institute.com and click on the GPRx Resource Guide.)

THE SKINNY ON FATS

Fats are needed by the body for serotonin production as well. In other words, fats are good for those battling depression.

You may be scratching your head and saying to yourself, *I thought fats were bad for you.* I don't blame you for feeling that way. Fats have gotten a bad rap ever since a pair of influential books were released in the 1990s. *The Pritikin Principle* by Nathan Pritikin and *The Ornish Diet* by Dean Ornish, M.D., backed up by zillions of follow-up stories and articles in the mainstream media, delivered the message that fat is something that you absolutely, positively have to avoid. Pritikin and Ornish preached the gospel of low-fat, high-carbohydrate diets, and they found millions of adherents, especially women believing they would be as thin as a Parisian supermodel if they dipped low-fat cookies into no-fat (or skim) milk. Then there was that woman with spiked platinum hair named Susan Powter who pleaded with TV viewers to "stop the insanity" because "it's fat that's making you fat!"

Girls in my high school nodded in agreement and gobbled up anything with the magic words "fat-free" or "reduced fat" on the packaging: cheese, crackers, cookies, yogurt, and ice cream. They studied salad-dressing labels as if they were the Dead Sea Scrolls, and they were obsessed with fat grams. I knew classmates who became borderline anorexic because of their fat phobia.

Although they put up nice fronts in the hallways, I bet that deep down they felt dispirited and despondent. When the body doesn't receive enough fat in the diet, less serotonin is produced, which only exacerbates feelings of depression and anxiety.

"Those who possess enough will power to remain fat-free for any length of time develop a variety of health problems including low energy, difficulty in concentration, *depression*, weight gain, and mineral deficiencies," wrote Mary Enig, Ph.D., and Sally Fallon in *Nourishing Traditions* (emphasis added).[5]

In my view, low-fat diets fail to distinguish between the so-called "good fats" in food (including olive and flaxseed oils, tropical oils such as coconut oil, and fish oils) and the "bad fats" (hydrogenated and processed oils found in margarine and most packaged goods). We need certain fats in our diet to provide a concentrated source of energy and source material for neurotransmitters in the brain, cell membranes, and various hormones. Fats also provide satiety; without them, we would be hungry within minutes of finishing a meal.

The problem with the standard American diet is that people eat too many of the wrong foods containing the wrong fats and not enough of the right foods with the right fats. The wrong fats are mainly hydrogenated and partially hydrogenated fats found in processed foods, as well as oils high in omega-6 fats such as soy, cottonseed, safflower, and corn oil, which fill cupboards and refrigerators in homes from Portland, Maine, to Portland, Oregon. Hydrogenated and partially hydrogenated fats are part of sugarcoated flakes for breakfast, a glazed doughnut at break time, fried corn chips and chocolate chip cookies for lunch, and breaded fried chicken nuggets for dinner.

When it comes to eating the right fats, I'm referring to a wide range of foods, including salmon, lamb, and goat meat; dairy products derived from goat's milk, sheep's milk, and cow's milk from grass-fed animals; and flaxseeds, walnuts, olives, macadamia nuts, and avocados. As for cooking, the top two fats and oils on my list are extra virgin coconut and olive oils, which are beneficial to the body's overall health. I urge you to cook with extra virgin coconut oil, which is a near-miracle food that few people have ever heard of. The medium-chain fatty acids in coconut oil are absorbed quickly by the tissues and converted to energy, which will give anyone battling a blue mood a lift.

Coconut oil is packed with antioxidants and reduces the body's need for vitamin E. You can tell which oil is better by comparing how fast canola oil or safflower oil becomes rancid when sitting at room temperature. Coconut oil shows no signs of rancidity even after a year at room temperature.

When moms heat up or fry food these days, however, they usually pour safflower, corn, or soybean oil (any of which may be partially hydrogenated) into the pan. In the process of hydrogenation, hydrogen gas is injected into the oil under high pressure to make the oil solid at room temperature, which prevents the oil from becoming rancid too quickly. Adulterating the oil carries a price, since the hydrogenation process produces trans-fatty acids, also known as trans fat.

Trans fat has recently become a household phrase since the Food and Drug Administration, beginning in 2006, required new Nutritional Facts labels on all foods to include information stating the amount of trans fat in that particular food. Trans fats are artery-clogging fats produced by heating liquid vegetable oils in the presence of hydrogen to make them solid at room temperature—a process known as *hydrogenation.*

Food manufacturers routinely utilize hydrogenated oil in their manufacturing plants, which means that trans fats are found in nearly all of our processed foods—foods that God definitely did *not* create. I'm talking about frozen pizza, ice cream, potato chips, cookie dough, white bread, dinner rolls, snack foods, doughnuts, candy, salad dressing, margarine—the list is endless. Why do food producers employ so much chemistry? Because it allows them to produce a more competitively priced product with a longer shelf life. Commercially prepared fried foods, like French fries and onion rings, also contain gobs of trans fat.

While oils and foods with trans fat should be eliminated from your diet, I can assure you that fats and oils created by God—as you would expect—are fats you want to include in your diet.

DEALING WITH CARBS

The third and final macronutrient is carbohydrates, which, by definition, are the sugars and starches contained in plant foods. Sugars and starches, like fats, are not bad for you, but the problem is that the standard American diet includes way too many foods containing these carbohydrates. Sugar and its sweet relatives—high fructose corn syrup, sucrose, molasses, and maple syrup—are among the first ingredients listed in staples such as cereals, breads, buns, pastries, doughnuts, cookies, ketchup, and ice cream.

A high carbohydrate diet, we know from science, increases the brain's production of serotonin. Does that mean you've been granted carte blanche to enjoy chocolate-glazed doughnuts, cinnamon buns, and ice cream sundaes? No, since these examples of "refined" carbohydrates come from sugar, which tends to provide immediate—but temporary—relief to your mood and energy level. Once your sweet tooth has been satisfied, the sugar rush quickly wears off and brings you lower, in terms of mood, than before you started to lick that ice cream cone.

You'll be much better off eating complex carbohydrates such as organic whole grain cereals, breads, and pastas, as well as fruits and vegetables, which are low glycemic, high nutrient, and low in sugar. These complex carbohydrates are also high in B vitamins, which are used in nervous system function. Vitamin B_6, for example, plays a leading role in the brain chemical production of serotonin and dopamine, and studies have shown that people who are depressed have low levels of B_6. Excellent sources of B_6 include bananas, bell peppers, turnip greens, spinach, as well as fish and poultry. (The richest source of vitamin B_6 is yellowfin tuna, which is off the chart.)

Eating unrefined carbohydrate foods introduces fiber into your body. Fiber is the indigestible remnants of plant cells found in vegetables, fruits, whole grains, nuts, seeds, and beans. Fiber-rich foods take longer to break down and are partially indigestible, which means that as these foods work their way through the digestive tract, they absorb water and increase the elimination of fecal waste in the large intestine.

Good sources of fiber are berries, fruits with edible skins

(apples, pears, and grapes), citrus fruits, gluten-free whole grains (quinoa, millet, amaranth, buckwheat, and brown rice), green peas, carrots, cucumbers, zucchini, tomatoes, and baked or boiled unpeeled potatoes. Green leafy vegetables such as spinach are also fiber rich. Eating foods high in fiber will immediately improve your blood sugar levels by slowing the absorption of sugars into your bloodstream.

Refined carbohydrates such as white bread, sweets, soft drinks, and processed foods deplete the body of B vitamins. They also clog things up in the digestive tract, which can lay a foundation for diet-related diseases, including depression. A gut-friendly diet is key, especially in light of Dr. Michael Gershon's assertion that nerve cells in the gut—the "second brain"—affect our mood. Remember the last time you had constipation? I bet you weren't in a very good mood during that episode.

When someone is constipated, an impermeable layer of toxins lines the intestinal wall, preventing nutrients from getting to the rest of the body. The brain's production of neurotransmitters, like serotonin, shuts down. They don't call this feeling "down in the dumps" for nothing.

Everyone feels better after a bowel movement. To keep things moving in the digestive tract, stay away from foods with refined sugar, which is a disaccharide carbohydrate that feeds harmful bacteria in the gastrointestinal tract. Starches such as bread, pasta, rice, corn, and potatoes are disaccharide carbohydrates as well, which are more difficult to digest. The digestive system finds these type of carbohydrates to be the most difficult to break down. What happens in the digestive process is that some undigested carbohydrates remain undigested in the large intestine, where they feed the undesirable microorganisms. When unabsorbed carbohydrates camp out in the colon, they feed harmful bacteria and upset the balance of the intestinal flora—and leave you feeling depressed.

The result—gas and acids caused by bacterial fermentation—becomes a vicious cycle. Undigested carbohydrates encourage bacterial fermentation, and bacterial fermentation makes it more difficult for carbohydrates to be absorbed. As you continue eating disaccharide-rich foods, your body never has a chance to catch up—or get in a good mood.

Diana Schwarzbein, M.D., author of *The Schwarzbein Principle*, wrote, "To achieve level moods, you need to eat enough food and good fats to balance insulin and other hormones." Balanced insulin, comes from a balanced diet. "When insulin levels are kept too low (by exercising, not eating enough food, or eliminating carbohydrates), you can waste away and may suffer from depression, fatigue, insomnia, and osteoporosis."[6]

In *The Great Physician's Rx for Depression and Anxiety*, I recommend that you avoid eating sugar unnecessarily and cut back on your starches considerably. I know that avoiding sugar is easier said than done. Many people unwittingly eat sugar with every meal: breakfast cereals are frosted with sugar, break time is soda or coffee mixed with sugar and a Danish, lunch has its cookies and treats, and dinner could be sweet-and-sour ribs topped off with a sugary dessert. But all those sweets can turn your health sour!

Chewing your food well will greatly improve the digestion of carbohydrates. If people tease you about "inhaling" your food, then you're eating too fast. I recommend chewing each mouthful of food twenty-five to seventy-five times before swallowing. This advice may sound ridiculous, but I know that a conscious effort to chew food slowly ensures that plenty of digestive juices are added to the food as it begins to wind through the digestive tract. I can't emphasize enough the critical importance of chewing your food well when you are dealing with depression and anxiety.

THE TOP HEALING FOODS

I've discussed many healthy foods in this chapter so far, but the following are musts to brighten your mood:

1. **Grass-fed meats and wild-caught fish.** As you know, I advocate eating organically raised, grass-fed cattle, sheep, goats, buffalo, and venison that graze on nature's bountiful grasses, and fish caught in the wild like salmon, tuna, or sea bass. Fish with fins and scales caught from oceans and rivers are lean sources of protein and provide essential fatty acids in abundance. Supermarkets are stocking these types of foods in greater quantities these days, and of course they are found in natural food stores, fish markets, and specialty stores.

You must avoid certain unhealthy meats. I'm talking about breakfast links, bacon, lunch meats, ham, hot dogs, bratwurst, and other sausages. I have reasons for recommending that you stay away from meats like bacon and ham lunch meat. In all of my previous books, I've consistently pointed out that pork—America's "other white meat"—should be avoided because pigs were called "unclean" in Leviticus and Exodus. God created pigs as scavengers—animals that survive just fine on any farm slop or water swill tossed their way. Pigs have a simple stomach arrangement: whatever a pig eats goes down the hatch, straight into the stomach, and out the back door in four hours max. They'll even eat their own excrement, if hungry enough.

Even if you decide to keep eating commercial beef instead of the organic version, I absolutely urge you to stop eating pork. Read Leviticus 11 and Deuteronomy 14 to learn what God said about eating clean versus unclean animals, where Hebrew words used to describe unclean meats can be translated as "detestable," "foul" and "putrid," the same terms that describe human waste.

Please realize that not all sea life is healthy to eat. Shellfish and fish without fins and scales, such as catfish, shark, and eel, are also described in Leviticus 11 and Deuteronomy 14 as detestable, unclean meats. God called hard-shelled crustaceans such as lobster, crabs, shrimp, and clams unclean because they are "bottom feeders," content to sustain themselves on excrement from other fish. To be sure, this purifies water but does nothing for the health of their flesh.

Eating unclean foods fouls the body and could very well foul your mood. God declared these meats detestable because He understands the ramifications of eating them, and you should as well.

2. **Cultured dairy products from goats, cows, and sheep.** When I began following the diet of the Bible, I consumed cultured dairy products such as yogurt and kefir from organically produced goat's, sheep's, and cow's milk. One benefit of eating cultured dairy is the beneficial microorganisms they contain. These living

organisms contain something called "probiotics," which, by definition, are living, direct-fed microbials (DFMs) that promote the growth of beneficial bacteria in the intestines. The normal human gastrointestinal tract contains hundreds of different species of harmless or even friendly bacteria, otherwise known as intestinal flora. When an imbalance of these bacteria occurs, the result is often constipation or diarrhea.

One of the best ways to introduce probiotics into my diet was through cultured dairy products such as raw cultured milk in the form of fermented kefir. Dairy products derived from goat's milk and sheep's milk can be easier on stomachs than those from cows, although dairy products from organic or grass-fed cows can be excellent as well. Goat's milk is less allergenic because it does not contain the same complex proteins found in cow's milk. I'm also a huge fan of sheep's milk.

If you've been having digestive problems, and your "second brain" has trouble coping, I recommend you avoid consuming fluid dairy products, such as milk and ice cream, since they contain the milk sugar lactose. Instead, I recommend eating fermented or cultured dairy products such as yogurt, kefir, hard cheeses, cultured cream cheese, cottage cheese, and cultured cream. Those who are lactose intolerant—and many with digestive ailments are sensitive to lactose—can often stomach fermented dairy products because they contain little or no residual lactose, which is the type of sugar in milk that many find hard to digest.

3. **Cultured and fermented vegetables.** Raw cultured or fermented vegetables such as sauerkraut, pickled carrots, beets, or cucumbers

supply the body with probiotics as well. Although these fermented vegetables are often greeted with upturned noses at the dinner table, these foods help reestablish natural balance to our digestive system. Sauerkraut, for example, is brimming with vitamins, such as vitamin C, and contains almost four times the nutrients as unfermented cabbage. The lactobacilli in fermented vegetables contain digestive enzymes that help break down food and increase its digestibility. I urge you to sample sauerkraut or pickled beets, which are readily available in health food stores.

4. **A wide selection of fruits and vegetables.** Fruits and vegetables right from the fields are the nutritional antithesis of processed foods, which come off an assembly line at a factory or industrial bakery. Fruits and veggies contain compounds that work to detoxify the digestive gut. Plant foods are the best sources in nature for antioxidants, which neutralize toxic substances in the body known as *free radicals.*

The Great Physician's Rx for Depression and Anxiety calls for the judicious intake of fruit, which can have a wonderful healing effect on the body. (Remember the last time you sank your teeth into a delicious peach?) I don't recommend that you eat fruit on its own because of its high sugar content, however. Fruit should be consumed with fats and proteins, which will slow down the absorption of sugar.

Limit your consumption to two or three servings of fresh fruit daily, which can be consumed during snack time. For those with depression, I recommend blueberries, strawberries, raspberries, and grapes, fully ripened and organic. When it comes to keeping your stomach calm, I believe you should eat organic fruits and vegetables that have not been grown with pesticides or chemical fertilizers. Try to eat fruits and vegetables in season; no one enjoys eating rubbery, half-green tomatoes. I'm fine with using frozen produce, since that often represents the best option for healthy fruits and veggies in the winter months. In the case of berries and certain fruits, the difference between fresh and frozen is minimal.

5. **Soaked and sprouted seeds and grains.** Like fruits and vegetables, whole grains, seeds, nuts, and breads made with sprouted or sour-leavened grains promote elimination, provide energy and endurance, and calm nerves. *Whole grain* means the bran and germ are left on the grain during processing.

Don't forget that highly refined, nutrient-deficient grains (refined rice, breads, and cereals) and sugars give you a rush before dropping your mood lower. This means you should say good-bye to white bread, hello to sprouted or sour-leavened whole wheat, rye, or flaxseed breads. Say good-bye to white rice, hello to brown rice and other healthy grains such as amaranth, quinoa, millet, and buckwheat. Say good-bye to pasta made from white enriched flour, hello to sprouted grain or spelt pasta, quinoa, barley, or couscous.

6. **Nuts.** Many nuts contain omega-3 and omega-6 essential fatty acids as well as tryptophan, which can boost the brain's production of serotonin. Try to eat some nuts daily. Grabbing a handful of almonds, cashews, pecans, pistachios, pumpkin seeds,

Brazil nuts, and pine nuts is a fine way to start you down the road toward better health.

7. **Spices.** Several household spices in your cupboard may have mood-elevating properties. Ginger, the world's most widely cultivated spice, contains chemicals that inhibit toxic bacteria in the digestive tract while it promotes friendly bacteria, which is why this spice is effective in treating conditions ranging from constipation to diarrhea. Ginger reduces the total volume of gastric juices, says Paul Schulick, author of *Ginger: Common Spice & Wonder Drug.* "From all parts of the world, virtually every ethnomedical text citing ginger has lauded its wide range of benefits to the digestive system," asserts Schulick.[7]

8. **Water.** Water isn't a food, of course, but this calorie-free and sugar-free substance performs many vital tasks for the body, including the production of mood-elevating serotonin. Let me explain.

Actually, I'll let F. Batmanghelidj, M.D., author of *You're Not Sick, You're Thirsty!,* explain how dehydration contributes to depression. As you know, certain amino acids, such as tryptophan, must reach the brain so that neurotransmitters such as serotonin and dopamine can be produced in order to keep the body's mood upbeat. In certain circumstances, some amino acids that have to reach the brain cells don't get there in sufficient amounts or quickly enough to cope with the demand. "The two main causes of shortfall in the delivery of the primary materials are dehydration and the overuse of the respective amino acids in other capacities," according to Dr. Batmanghelidj wrote. "Dehydration causes problems with the transport process across the blood-brain barrier."[8]

What Dr. Batmanghelidj is saying is that water energizes the brain, which is like a water-wheel house. In other words, picture water passing through a water wheel, which produces hydro-electricity, and you have an idea of how water is the power source for the brain. "With dehydration, the level of energy generation in the brain is decreased. Many silent functions of the brain that depend on hydroelectric energy become inefficient. We recognize this inadequacy of function and call it depression."[9]

You should drink a minimum of eight glasses of water a day, or better yet, drink a half-ounce of water per pound of body weight. In other words, a 140-pound female needs to drink seventy ounces of water per day to stay hydrated. Water regulates the body temperature, carries nutrients and oxygen to the cells, cushions joints, protects organs and tissue, and removes toxins. Water provides the viscosity in blood and plasma, almost like the lubricating effects of oil in a high-powered engine. Water helps move nutrients to your cells and helps keep cholesterol levels down. Not drinking enough water is bad for your body and for your mental health.

Sure, you'll go to the bathroom more often, but is that so bad? Drinking plenty of water is a key element of the Great Physician's Rx for Depression and Anxiety Battle Plan (see page 74), so keep a water bottle close by and drink water before, during, and in between meals. I take hydration seriously even though I'm not battling depression. I set a forty-eight-ounce bottle of water on my office desk as a reminder to keep putting fluids into my system. My record for drinking water is one and one-quarter gallons of water in a day during a fast, but I won't reveal how many trips I made to the bathroom.

This seems like a good place to talk about this country's obsession with coffee, thanks to your neighborhood Starbucks. For those battling depression and anxiety, I urge you to stay away from coffee. Caffeine depletes the body of vitamin B_6 and can have a depressive effect in larger amounts. In a study, caffeine users reported significantly higher depression scores when compared to nondrinkers of caffeine. The higher the total caffeine intake, the more likely the subjects were to suffer from depression.[10]

Teas and herbal infusions (the latter beverage is made from herbs and spices, rather than the actual tea plant) are a better story altogether. My favorite tea blends contain green, black, or rooibos tea that come in a handy liquid pack. Even though I've never thought of myself as a tea-drinking type, my wife, Nicki, and I enjoy these tea blends with meals.

You'll find in my Great Physician's Rx for Depression and Anxiety Battle Plan (see page 74) that I recommend a cup of hot tea and honey with breakfast, dinner, and snacks. I also advise consuming freshly made iced tea, as tea can be consumed hot or steeped and iced. Please note that while herbal tea provides many great health benefits, nothing can replace pure water for hydration. Although you can safely and healthfully consume two to four cups per day of tea and herbal infusions, you still need to drink at least eight cups (or a half-ounce per pound of body weight) of pure water for all the good reasons I've described in this section.

PRACTICE FASTING ONCE A WEEK

Most people, when they read about a recommendation to fast, think that not eating for a length of time would make them *more* depressed, rather than lift their moods out of depressed depths.

Let me assure you that just the opposite will happen. *The Encyclopedia of Natural Healing* says that not only do people experience a tremendous sense of well-being and increased vitality when they come off a fast, but a fast can counteract depression and moodiness.[11] What a fast does is detoxify the body, allowing the organs and digestive tract to "reboot," so to speak. You give the body an opportunity to cleanse and heal itself. You feel better when you come off a fast, and when you feel better, your mood lifts. Fasting is inexpensive and can be done today.

While taking a sustained break from eating will improve your physical health and mental outlook in ways you can't understand, there's a spiritual side to fasting that must be addressed as well. When you fast and pray (two words that seem to go hand in hand in Scripture), you are pursuing God in your life and opening yourself to experiencing a renewed sense of well-being and dependence upon the Lord.

The Bible is full of references to fasting—seventy-four in all—and tells how spiritual giants such as David, Daniel, and Paul experienced periods of fasting before launching themselves into doing God's work. Isaiah 58:6, 8 says, "Is not this the kind of fasting I have chosen: . . . to set the oppressed free and break every yoke? . . . Then your light will break forth like the dawn, and your healing will quickly appear" (NIV).

So if you're feeling depressed, give fasting a try. I recommend starting with a one-day partial fast once a week. In this type of fast, you wake up in the morning and refrain from eating breakfast and lunch, as well as any snacks. Then you resume eating with a dinnertime meal. I've found that Thursdays or Fridays work best for me because the week is winding down and the weekend is coming up. For instance, I won't eat breakfast and lunch so that when I break my fast and eat dinner that night, my body has gone between eighteen and twenty hours without food or sustenance since I last ate dinner the night before.

The benefits are immediate: you'll feel great, lose weight, look younger, save money, save time, and become closer to the Lord.

What Not to Eat

When you're dealing with depression and anxiety, there are a number of foods that should never find a way onto your plate or into your hands. I call them "The Dirty Dozen." Some I've already discussed elsewhere in this chapter, while the rest are presented here with a short commentary:

1. **Processed meat and pork products.** These meats top my list because they are staples in the standard American diet and are extremely unhealthy because of the high amounts of sodium they contain, among other things.

The meats you must steer clear of are breakfast links, bacon, lunch meats, ham, bratwurst, and other sausages because they introduce pathogenic organisms and toxins into the bloodstream, and because God called them "detestable" and "unclean" in Leviticus and Exodus. These processed meats also contain additives like nitrates that were introduced during the curing process. Nitrates can convert into nitrite, which can form into nitrosamines, powerful cancer-causing chemicals.

2. Shellfish and fish without fins and scales, such as catfish, shark, and eel. Am I saying au revoir and sayonara to lobster thermidor and shrimp tempura? That's what I'm saying.

3. Hydrogenated oils. Be aware that the hydrogenated or partially hydrogenated fats in processed foods—from commercial cakes, pastries, and desserts to just about every wrapped-in-plastic item sold in a neighborhood convenience store—are bad for you. If you can hop off the junk food bandwagon and leave all those hydrogenated oils behind, your depression could be in your rearview mirror.

4. Artificial sweeteners. Aspartame (found in NutraSweet and Equal), saccharine (Sweet'N Low), and sucralose (Splenda), which are chemicals several hundred times sweeter than sugar, should be completely avoided by those dealing with depression and anxiety. Simply put, these are not foods at all, but combinations of artificial chemicals that may lead to serious problems for those who consume them.

H. J. Roberts, M.D., said in his book *Aspartame Disease: An Ignored Epidemic*, that aspartame depletes serotonin, and you know what happens when the brain doesn't produce enough of this neurotransmitter: mood swings, anxiety, and depression. My friend, Dr. Joe Mercola of the influential Mercola.com Web site, says that aspartame accounts for more than 75 percent of the adverse reactions to food additives reported to the FDA. We're talking about headaches, dizziness, numbness, nausea, and other digestive difficulties. Bottom line: these blue, pink, and yellow packets contain questionable compounds that don't deserve a place in your cupboard or your cup of coffee.

5. **White flour.** White flour isn't a problematic chemical like artificial sweeteners, but it's virtually worthless and not healthy for you because of the processing that goes into turning wheat into white flour.

After wheat is harvested, the wheat stalks are trucked to flour mills and rinsed with various chemical bleaches that sound like a vocabulary test from high school biology class: nitrogen oxide, chlorine, chloride, nitrosyl, and benzoyl peroxide. The result is that half of the healthy fatty acids are lost in the milling process, as well as the wheat germ and bran, which contain vitamins and fiber. By removing most of the naturally occurring nutrients and adding chemicals and a few isolated and synthetic vitamins and minerals, we've managed to take a healthy food that's been on families' tables for centuries—usually in the form of bread, pasta, or baked goods—and turn it into one of the most highly allergenic, difficult-to-digest substances.

The healthier alternative is eating whole wheat bread and other whole grain products made from unprocessed whole grain flour.

6. **White sugar.** Sugar comes in so many forms that it's hard to keep track of the names used for it these days. If the food label utilizes descriptions like corn syrup, high-fructose corn syrup, sucrose, corn sweeteners, sorghum syrup, or fruit juice concentrate, you're essentially eating sugar.

7. **Soft drinks.** These are nothing more than liquefied sugar. A twenty-ounce Coke or Pepsi is the equivalent of eating fifteen teaspoons of sugar. Diet drinks loaded with artificial sweeteners are even worse, as noted in point number 4.

8. **Corn syrup.** Another version of sugar and just as bad for you, if not worse.

9. **Pasteurized homogenized skimmed milk.** Like I said, whole organic, nonhomogenized milk is better and cultured milk from grass-fed cows, sheeps, and goats is best.

10. **Hydrolyzed soy protein.** Hydrolyzed soy protein is found in imitation meat products such as imitation crab. In his book *Excitotoxins: The Taste That Kills,* author Russell L. Blaylock, M.D., explained how monosodium glutamate (MSG), hydrolyzed vegetable protein, aspartame, aspartate, and other chemicals found in our foods are examples of excitotoxins, which are substances that overexcite neurons to the point of cell damage and, eventually, cell death. Food manufacturers add these chemicals, Dr. Blaylock points out, because they stimulate the taste cells in the tongue, thereby enhancing the taste of the

food. Don't take a chance with fouling your health by eating hydrolyzed soy protein.

11. **Artificial flavors and colors.** These are never good for you under the best of circumstances, and certainly not when you're battling depression.

12. **Excessive alcohol.** Alcohol is a natural depressant, or downer, because it reduces brain activity. If you are depressed *before* you start drinking, several drinks will have you feeling even more dejected faster than you can say, "I'll have another."

EAT: WHAT FOODS ARE EXTRAORDINARY, AVERAGE, OR TROUBLE?

I've prepared a comprehensive list of foods that are ranked in descending order based on their health-giving qualities. Foods at the top of the list are healthier than those at the bottom. The best foods to serve and eat are what I call "Extraordinary." These are foods which God created for us to eat and will give you the best chance to live a long and happy life. If you are battling depression and anxiety, it's best to consume foods from the extraordinary category more than 75 percent of the time.

Foods in the Average category should make up less than 25 percent of your daily diet. These foods should be consumed sparingly. Foods in the Trouble category should be consumed with extreme caution. If you're dealing with persistent depression, you should avoid these foods completely.

For a complete listing of Extraordinary, Average, and Trouble Foods, visit www.BiblicalHealthInstitute.com.

℞ THE GREAT PHYSICIAN'S RX FOR DEPRESSION AND ANXIETY: EAT TO LIVE

- *Eat only foods God created.*

- *Eat foods in a form that is healthy for the body.*

- *Consume foods high in omega-3 fatty acids such as wild-caught fish and organic eggs.*

- *Consume foods high in fiber.*

- *Increase consumption of raw fruits and vegetables.*

- *Increase consumption of leafy greens, grass-fed red meat, and high omega-3 eggs.*

- *Practice fasting one day per week.*

- *Drink eight or more glasses of pure water per day.*

- *Avoid foods high in sugar.*

- *Avoid foods containing hydrogenated oils.*

Take Action

To learn how to incorporate the principles of eating to
live into your daily lifestyle, please turn to page 74 for
the Great Physician's Rx for Depression and Anxiety
Battle Plan.

KEY #2

Supplement Your Diet with Whole Food
Nutritionals, Living Nutrients, and Superfoods

We know that omega-3 and omega-6 essential fatty acids (EFAs) play a critical role in the function of the central nervous system, including the production of brain chemicals recognized as neurotransmitters. We also know that nutritional shortcuts have been taken regarding today's commercially raised beef, chicken, and fish as well as fruits and vegetables grown in nutrient-barren soils. Bottom line: this is just one example of how our diets aren't doing what they're supposed to do—keep us in optimal health.

That's why many people, including myself, look to nutritional supplements to bridge the gap. When it comes to depression and anxiety, laboratory and clinical studies suggest that deficiencies in omega-3 and omega-6 fatty acids, any of the B vitamins, and vitamin D cause fatigue and depression. Supplementing your diet with whole food nutritionals containing these nutrients is a key part of the Great Physician's prescription for those with depression and anxiety.

A go-to supplement, the one topping my list, is omega-3 cod liver oil. Cod liver oil contains four nutrients that hardly any of us get enough of: eicosapentaenoic acid (EPA), docosahexaenoic acid (DHA), vitamin A, and vitamin D. EPA and DHA are long-chain polyunsaturated fats known as omega-3 fatty acids, which the brain uses to produce neurotransmitters like serotonin and which also help nerve cells communicate with each other, which is essential in maintaining good mental health.

"Levels of omega-3 fatty acids were found to be measurably low, and the ratio of omega-6 to omega-3 fatty acids were particularly high in a study of patients with depression," according to researchers at the University of Maryland Medical Center. "In a study of people with depression those who ate a healthy diet consisting of fatty fish two or three times per week for five years experienced a significant reduction in feelings of depression and hostility."[1] In addition, a Harvard study showed that fish oil supplements helped modify the mood swings of patients suffering from manic depression.[2]

Many folks, for whatever reason, aren't able to eat fatty fish two or three times a week (and for five years!), so here's where supplementation comes in. I recommend taking between one teaspoon and one tablespoon of omega-3 cod liver oil each day to receive those much-needed omega-3 fatty acids. Sure, you may have to hold your nose, but if school kids in Reykjavik, Iceland, have no problem taking this supplement known for its fishy odor and taste, then you shouldn't either. Besides, there are some excellent brands that come in lemon, mint, and other flavors, as well as capsules.

Cod liver oil from Norwegian or Icelandic cod also contains high amounts of vitamin D. Canadian researchers at Mt. Sinai Hospital in Toronto believe that vitamin D relieves depression after a study showed that patients suffering from depression improved when their vitamin D levels increased.[3]

I added omega-3 cod liver oil to my daily diet ten years ago when I was making my recovery from a two-year illness that led to major episodes of depression. Now I'm to the point where I can drink the stuff right out of the bottle.

If you can't stomach the thought of sipping omega-3 cod liver oil, you can now take this important nutrient in easy-to-swallow liquid capsules.

WHOLE FOOD MULTIVITAMINS

Taking multivitamins made from "whole food" sources—I'll get into that in a minute—is a great way to ensure you're getting enough B vitamins, which are generally credited in medical circles with having favorable effects on mental health and depression. "The B-complex vitamins are essential to mental and emotional well-being," says Nancy Schimelpfening, a health columnist for the About.com Web site. "They cannot be stored in our bodies, so we depend entirely on our daily diet to supply them. B vitamins are destroyed by alcohol, refined sugars, nicotine, and caffeine, so it is no surprise that many people may be deficient in these."[4]

Keep in mind that alcohol and refined sugars were part of the "Dirty Dozen" in Key #1, and I didn't recommend smoking, or drinking excess caffeinated coffee either. At any rate, a whole food multivitamin will supply you with a well-rounded source of B vitamins, such as:

- B_1, which the brain uses to help convert glucose, or
  blood sugar, into fuel. A lack of B_1 can lead to
  depression, anxiety, and even thoughts of suicide.[5]

- B_6, which is needed in the brain's manufacture of the neurotransmitters serotonin and dopamine.
- B_{12}, which is important to red blood cell formation. A deficiency can cause mood swings and paranoia.

B vitamins are part of good whole food multivitamins, which contain different compounds such as organic acids, antioxidants, and key nutrients. Whole food multivitamins, or "living" supplements, are more costly to produce since the ingredients—fruits, vegetables, sea vegetables, seeds, spices, vitamins and minerals, etc.—are put through a fermentation process similar to the digestive process of the body, but they are well worth the extra money.

The best multivitamins are produced from raw materials by adding vitamins and minerals to a living probiotic culture. If you're scratching your head and saying, "Huh?" let me explain. Multivitamins are produced in several different ways. Some are derived from vegetable, mineral, or animal sources such as cod liver oil, wheat germ oil, or yeast. Other multivitamins are derived from processing that extracts vitamins from fish liver oil, soybeans, and other natural sources.

The most common form of multivitamins, however, is synthetically produced in a chemist's lab and is also the cheapest to produce. If you see ingredients such as sucrose, cornstarch, thiamine mononitrate, pyridoxine hydrochloride, ascorbic acid, or sodium metasilicate listed, your multivitamin is produced from synthetic materials. Synthetic multivitamins are never going to be as good or potent as ones produced from natural sources; studies show that synthetically made vitamins are 50 to 70 percent less biologically active than vitamins created from natural sources.

Whole food multivitamins come packaged in different varieties: tablets and capsules are the most common; powders and liquids are less widespread. I prefer caplets as a good delivery system to ensure that the nutrients get where they need to go.

Probiotics and Digestive Enzymes

Since how you feel in your gut is also related to your mental and behavioral health as well as mood, I recommend taking probiotics and digestive enzyme supplements because of the way they help the digestive tract. Probiotics are friendly microorganisms that increase your ability to absorb nutrients from food while promoting the growth of beneficial bacteria in the intestines—your "second brain."

Probiotics in dietary supplement form are a great way to reintroduce beneficial microorganisms into your digestive tract, which can improve bowel and immune system function, increase nutrient absorption, and detoxify the body and its organs. I think the best probiotics are the ones that contain lactic-acid bacteria, soil-based organisms, and beneficial yeasts, which are room-temperature stable and do not require refrigeration as most common probiotic supplements do.

Digestive enzymes are complex proteins involved in the digestive process. Enzymes are the body's day laborers, the ones responsible for synthesizing, delivering, and eliminating the unbelievable number of ingredients and chemicals that your body uses during the waking hours. When the body produces enzymes, their job is to stimulate chemical changes in the foods passing through the gut. The pancreas, which takes a lead role in producing digestive enzymes for the body, has to keep up by producing pancreatic enzymes.

Junk-food diets, fast chewing, and eating on the run contribute to the body's inability to produce adequate enzyme production and the subsequent malabsorption of food. One could eat more raw food in its natural, unprocessed state, but that isn't always possible, as I can attest when I travel or have a heavy social schedule. The last thing you want to eat when you have digestive problems is fried foods, because items like fried chicken and French fries must be cooked in oil at higher temperatures than the boiling point, which damages fats and destroys all enzymes.

So, if you're having trouble finding a way to eat enough raw, fresh foods like bananas, avocados, seeds, nuts, grapes, and other natural foods, then take plant-based digestive enzymes to ease matters in your digestive tract. Digestive enzymes are available at your local natural food store, and you can find recommended brands by visiting www.BiblicalHealthInstitute.com and clicking on the GPRx Resource Guide.

Adaptogenic Herbs

I'm not a huge believer in pinning your hopes on St. John's wort for treating depression, but I am impressed with two other herbs: the eastern Indian herb *Ashwaghandha* and the Russian herb *Rhodiola rosea*. Ashwaghandha root has been used for centuries in

Ayurvedic medicine, the traditional medicine system originating in India. Rhodiola rosea, also known as Golden Root, is a perennial plant that grows in dry, sandy ground at high altitudes in the arctic areas of Siberia. This herb has been used in Russian traditional medicine for relieving anxiety and depression for hundreds of years.

Ashwaghandha and Rhodiola rosea are adaptogens, which are endurance enhancers. In various research studies, Ashwaghandha and Rhodiola rosea, when mixed into hot water, like tea, or taken in supplement form, have been found to:

- benefit overall health and control stress-related weight gain,
- revitalize metabolic processes associated with restlessness and fatigue,
- promote emotional well being,
- regulate and balance body organs for increased physical and mental rejuvenation, and
- support blood sugar and cholesterol levels already within the normal range.

Rhodiola rosea, from everything I've heard and read, is an absolute superstar when it comes to depression. In an open clinical trial of Rhodiola rosea's ability to alleviate depression symptoms, 65 percent of those who participated in the trial said the extract was effective in reducing or removing symptoms of depression.[6] Said the authors of *The Rhodiola Revolution*, "Since the 1990s, renewed interest in reducing psychological stress has pushed Rhodiola rosea to the forefront of scientific exploration. In all of the studies to date, the herb has significantly lessened mental stress and anxiety while enhancing mood and intellectual performance."[7]

WHOLE FOOD FIBER

My final recommendation is for a whole food fiber supplement that supplies your body with a highly usable, vegetarian source of dietary fiber. A whole food fiber supplement can counteract the refined foods that glut the stomach and stop you up.

When searching for a fiber product that's right for you, choose a brand that is made from organic seeds, grains, and legumes that are fermented or sprouted for ease of digestion. One of the best ways to consume whole food fiber is to take it first thing in the morning and just before bed. Taking a daily dose of whole food fiber is great to keep that "second brain" healthy. (For a list of recommended whole food fiber products, visit www. BiblicalHealthInstitute.com and click on the GPRx Resource Guide.)

℞ THE GREAT PHYSICIAN'S RX FOR DEPRESSION AND ANXIETY: SUPPLEMENT YOUR DIET WITH WHOLE FOOD NUTRITIONALS AND LIVING NUTRIENTS

- *Consume one to three teaspoons or three to nine capsules of omega-3 cod liver oil per day.*

- *Take a whole food living multivitamin.*

- *Be sure to introduce beneficial microorganisms (probiotics) into your diet daily, as well as digestive enzymes with each meal.*

- *Adopt adaptogenic herbs such as Ashwaghandha and Rhodiola rosea into your supplementation plan.*

- *Take a whole food fiber supplement twice per day, morning and evening.*

Take Action

To learn how to incorporate the principles of supplementing your diet with whole food nutritionals, living nutrients and superfoods, please turn to page 74 for the Great Physician's Rx for Depression and Anxiety Battle Plan.

Key #3

Practice Advanced Hygiene

The poster boy for obsessive-compulsive disorder would be Howard Hughes, America's first billionaire who was consumed with designing airplanes, dating starlets, producing movies, and fighting microbial infection. As the biopic film, *The Aviator,* demonstrated, Hughes was a germ-a-phobe who'd wash his hands until they bled.

I fly in and out of airports probably forty-eight weeks a year, so I often think of Howard Hughes when I visit an airport restroom. It's absolutely brutal watching guys do their thing at the urinals and fail to wash up afterward, but after reading a San Diego State University study about the cleanliness of airline bathrooms, I'm thinking about staying in my seat until I land.

San Diego State biology professor Scott Kelley took a small but scientific sampling of airline cleanliness by sending observers to swab surfaces at ten different places aboard various flights. They took biological evidence not only from armrests and tray tables, but toilet seats and handles, sinks, floors, unused paper towels, and doorknobs coming in and out of the planes' bathrooms.

After studying the microbial scuzz under a microscope, he determined that airline bathrooms were flying germ farms. "It was worse than a fraternity house in there," professor Kelley declared, referring to the toilets forward and aft. "I can't think of a more diverse area [of bacterial contamination]."[1] He discovered opportunistic pathogens like *Streptococcus, Staphylococcus, Cornybacterium, Proprionibacterium,* and *Kocuria* in his study published in the *Journal of Applied Microbiology.*[2]

Kelley said the situation doesn't warrant wearing surgical gloves the next time you board a flight, but he mentioned that whenever he flies and uses the facilities, he washes his hands well and uses a paper towel to open the lavatory door as he leaves. The bathroom knob was the nastiest part of the plane, the researcher said.

While life's too short to become paranoid like Howard Hughes, it's a biological fact that our hands pick up germs from everything we touch: lavatory doors, doorknobs, countertops, money, telephones, shopping carts, pens, and pencils. Chuck Gerba, a University of Arizona environmental-microbiology professor, says that 80 percent of infections, from colds and flu viruses to food-borne diseases, are spread through contact with hands and surfaces.

Germs *love* the hands, because once they establish a beachhead on your fingertips and under your nails, it's only a matter of time before you touch your lips, rub your eyes, scratch your nose, or itch your ears. Dr. Gerba, known in the media as Dr. Germ, says that the average adult touches his or her face one to three times every five minutes.[3] When—not if—the hand touches part of your face, bacteria are successfully transferred from your fingertips to one of these portals to your body. In the time it takes to sneeze, your body's immune system comes under attack. When viruses invade the respiratory system, the body launches a counterattack that lays waste to outside intruders or repairs any infected bodily organs.

This is noteworthy because Key #3 of the Great Physician's

prescription, "Practice Advanced Hygiene," can protect your body from being the recipient of a garden variety of bacteria, allergens, environmental toxins, and viruses that are transferred from one part of the body to the other. In addition, germs affect the health of the gut—think parasites—and the gut affects the brain, so for those battling depression and anxiety, it's vital to practice advanced hygiene.

I've been taking proactive steps to protect my digestive tract and immune system by following an advanced hygiene protocol life for more than ten years, and the results have been dramatic: no depressing moods, no lingering head colds, no nagging sinus infections, and no acute respiratory illnesses to speak of for many years. I follow a program first developed by an Australian scientist, Kenneth Seaton, Ph.D., who discovered that ear, nose, throat, and skin problems could be linked to the fact that humans touch their noses, eyes, and mouths with germ-carrying fingernails throughout the day. "Germs don't fly, they hitchhike," Dr. Seaton declared, and he's right.

Dr. Seaton estimates that once you pick up hitchhiking germs, they hibernate and hide around the fingernails, no matter how short you keep them trimmed. I know this stuff isn't pleasant dinnertime conversation, but practicing advanced hygiene has become an everyday habit for me.

Since I'm aware that 90 percent of germs take up residence around my fingernails, I use a creamy, semisoft soap rich in essential oils. Each morning and evening, I dip both of my hands into the tub of semisoft soap and dig my fingernails into the cream. Then I work the special cream around the tips of fingers, cuticles, and fingernails for fifteen to thirty seconds. When I'm finished, I rinse my hands under running water, lathering them for fifteen seconds before rinsing. After my hands are clean, I take another dab of semisoft soap and wash my face.

My next step involves a procedure that I call a "facial dip." I fill my washbasin or a clean large bowl with warm but not hot water. When enough water is in the basin, I add one to two tablespoons of regular table salt and two eyedroppers of a mineral-based facial solution into the cloudy water. I mix everything up with my hands and then I bend over and dip my face into the cleansing matter, opening my eyes several times to allow the membranes to be cleansed. After coming up for air, I dunk my head a second time and blow bubbles through my nose. "Sink snorkeling," I call it.

My final two steps of advanced hygiene involve the application of very diluted drops of hydrogen peroxide and minerals into my ears for thirty to sixty seconds to cleanse the ear canal, followed by brushing my teeth with an essential oil tooth solution to cleanse my teeth, gums, and mouth of unhealthy germs. (For more information on my favorite advanced hygiene products, visit www.BiblicalHealthInstitute and click on the GPRx Resource Guide.)

Brushing your teeth well and regularly practicing advanced hygiene involves discipline; you have to remind yourself to do it until it becomes an ingrained habit. I find it easier to follow these steps in the morning when I'm freshly awake than later in the evening when I'm tired and bleary-eyed—although I do my best to practice advanced hygiene morning and evening and hardly ever miss. Either way, I know it only takes three minutes or so to complete all of the advanced hygiene steps, and those might be the best three minutes a day for maintaining your health.

A Primer on Washing Your Hands

1. Wet your hands with warm water. It doesn't have to be anywhere near scalding hot.

2. Apply plenty of soap into the palms of both hands. The best soap to use is a semisoft soap that you can dig your fingernails into.

3. Rub your hands vigorously together and scrub all the surfaces. Pay attention to the skin between the fingers and work the soap into the fingernails.

4. Rub and scrub for fifteen to thirty seconds, or about the time it takes to slowly sing "Happy Birthday."

5. Rinse well and dry your hands on a paper towel or clean cloth towel. If you're in a public restroom, it's a good idea to turn off the running water with the towel in your hand. An even *better* idea is to use that same towel to open the door, since that door handle is the first place that nonwashers touch after they've gone to the bathroom.

6. Keep waterless sanitizers in your purse or wallet in case soap and water are not available in the public restroom. These towelettes, although not ideal, are better than nothing.

When to Wash Your Hands

- after you go to the bathroom
- before and after you insert and remove contact lenses
- before and after food preparation
- before you eat
- after you sneeze, cough, or blow your nose
- after cleaning up after your pet
- after handling money
- after changing a diaper
- after wiping a child's nose
- after handling garbage
- after cleaning your toilets
- after shaking a bunch of hands
- after shopping at the supermarket
- after attending an event at a public theater
- before and after sexual intercourse

R THE GREAT PHYSICIAN'S RX FOR DEPRESSION AND ANXIETY: PRACTICE ADVANCED HYGIENE

- *Dig your fingers into a semisoft soap with essential oils and wash your hands regularly, paying special attention to removing germs from underneath your fingernails.*

- *Cleanse your nasal passageways and the mucous membranes of the eyes daily by performing a facial dip.*

- *Cleanse the ear canals at least twice per week.*

- *Use an essential oil–based tooth solution daily to remove germs from the teeth, gums, and mouth.*

Take Action

To learn how to incorporate the principles of practicing advanced hygiene into your daily lifestyle, please turn to page 74 for the Great Physician's Rx for Depression and Anxiety Battle Plan.

KEY #4

Condition Your Body
with Exercise and Body Therapies

Depression has a way of making you feel powerless to do anything to break life's vicious cycle. To paraphrase New York Yankee great Yogi Berra, "Depression is 90 percent mental. The other half is physical."

When it comes to exercise, many with depression and anxiety disorders have another New Yorker phrase on their lips: *fuggedaboutit.* Too much effort. Too depressing. Even though a walk around the park is often the *last* thing depressed people feel like doing, there's good evidence that exercise is beneficial for mild to moderate depression.

Indeed, exercise is an excellent antidote to any stress and anxiety in your life. Huffing and puffing on a treadmill, for example, blows off steam like a teakettle. Walking in the quiet of the morning helps you prepare for your day by giving you time to think about your schedule—what you need to accomplish, whom you need to call, and what appointments you need to keep. An energetic tennis game stimulates the mind and provides a mental break from reading reports and crunching numbers. A stroll in a park or walk down a golf fairway provides a welcome change of scenery from whatever's bothering you. Doing yard work or going on a spring-cleaning binge around the house gives you a sense of accomplishment.

Whatever its form, exercise is a superior way to slice stress from your life for these reasons:

1. Exercising is a leisure pursuit that by its very nature lowers anxiety, reduces stress, and improves mood.
2. Although exercising adds another time commitment to our lives, it doesn't seem to create *more* stress.

David Nieman, an Appalachian State University researcher, put a control group of "stressed-out" women (as determined by psychological testing) on a brisk walking program. After a month of walking, he tested them against a sedentary control group and found that the walking women "maintained an elevated mood."[1]

Theories abound for why this is so, but most researchers point to the endorphins and other feel-good chemicals released by the body during a workout. Sports medicine psychologist Dr. Jim Loehr says that the release of these powerful chemicals (such as catecholamine, adrenaline, noradrenaline, hydrocortisone, and glucocorticoid) causes immune cells to be released and protective chemicals to flood the cardiovascular system, protecting the body against illness and lifting mood. I tend to think of fitness as a therapeutic "time out" that builds the mood and helps people ward off stress.

"Exercise isn't a cure for depression or anxiety," say the doctors from the Mayo Clinic. "But its psychological and physical benefits can improve your symptoms. Exercising may be the last thing you think you can do, but you can overcome the inertia."[2]

I have a background in physical fitness, having been a personal trainer at one time. If you were my client, having been informed by your doctor that you have depression, I would start you with *functional fitness.* This form of gentle exercise will raise your heartbeat, strengthen the body's core muscles, and exercise the cardiovascular system through the performance of real-life activities in real-life positions.

Functional fitness can be done with no equipment or by employing dumbbells, mini-trampolines, and stability balls. You can find functional fitness classes and equipment at gyms around the country, including LA Fitness, Bally Total Fitness, and local YMCAs. You'll be asked to perform squats with feet apart, feet together, and one back with the other forward. You'll be asked to do reaching lunges, push-ups against a wall, and "supermans" that involve lying on the floor and lifting up your right arm while lifting your left leg into a fully extended position. What you *won't* be asked to perform are high-impact exercises like those found in pulsating aerobics classes. (For more information on functional fitness, visit www.BiblicalHealthInstitute.com.)

Your goal should be to exercise at least twenty to thirty minutes three times a week. Four or five times a week is better, and six days a week is best.

LET THE SUN SHINE IN

The only thing better than exercise would be exercising in the sun.

Seriously. Those who treat depression have noticed for a long time that people complain the most about feeling depressed during the late fall and winter months, when sunlight is scarce.

Doctors even have a name for it: seasonal affective disorder (SAD). As someone who lives in Florida—the Sunshine State—year-round, I can hardly imagine what it's like to live in the Northeast and Pacific Northwest, where gray skies are the norm during winter. Not seeing the sun for days or weeks at a time has to contribute to an air of gloominess.

Sunlight is a critical contributor to vitamin D in the body. Remember how I mentioned in Key #2 that those with depression need vitamin D? Actually, vitamin D is not a vitamin but a critical hormone that regulates the health of more than thirty different tissues and organs, including the brain. One of the best ways to receive this beneficial hormone is by sitting outside in bright sunshine. Getting sunlight is extremely important for our bodies because of the way our skin synthesizes vitamin D from the ultraviolet rays of sunlight. The National Institutes of Health (NIH) state that all you need is ten to fifteen minutes of sunlight for vitamin D synthesis to occur.

SLEEP TIME

"How are you sleeping these days?"

That's one of the first questions a doctor will ask you if you come into his office complaining of not having that old pep. Depression and anxiety take a toll on how much nighttime rest you get. Sometimes depression, and the antidepressant medications you're taking for it, prompts you to sleep too much. More often—85 percent of the time, according to researchers—those suffering from depression battle insomnia or wake up too early in the morning. Either way, depression and anxiety sufferers often get out of bed feeling totally unrefreshed.

Getting more sleep can have a huge impact on your mood, but when you're feeling down, it's difficult to "switch off" depressive or anxious thoughts or wind down after a long day. Overcrowded schedules, the desire to accomplish one more thing before retiring, and too much stimulation from watching TV in bed or late at night keeps the mind working overtime.

Sure, it would be easy to say, "Just go to bed earlier," but I have a different tack. An hour of sleep *before* midnight is worth four hours of sleep *after* midnight, according to Dr. Joseph Mercola, founder of the Mercola.com Web site. Getting more sleep won't happen overnight (no pun intended), so I would start by retiring fifteen minutes earlier than usual and seeing how that goes before increasing that to thirty minutes earlier than usual. This may involve some discipline with the TV: most people stay up late to watch ESPN's SportsCenter, Letterman, or Leno. If you can't bear the thought of missing your favorite show, then TiVo it for viewing another time.

How much sleep do you need? The goal should be eight hours, which would be around an hour more than what the average American adult receives these days, according to the National Sleep Foundation. Eight hours is the magic number because when people are allowed to "sleep out" and wake up when they want to under controlled laboratory conditions, they generally sleep eight hours in a twenty-four-hour period. This twenty-four-hour period, called the *circadian rhythm*, mirrors the twenty-four hours it takes for the earth to rotate on its axis.

Sleep is good for the body and good for your mental health. William Shakespeare wasn't too far off when he wrote four hundred years ago, "Sleep that knits up the ravel'd sleave of care . . . chief nourisher in life's feast."

In addition to proper sleep, the body needs a time of rest every seven days to recharge its batteries. This is accomplished by taking a break from the rat race on Saturday or Sunday. God created the earth and the heavens in six days and rested on the seventh, giving you an example and a reminder that you need to take a break from your labors. Otherwise, you're a prime candidate for burnout and depression.

A WARM SPOT

Baths, showers, steam rooms, saunas, washings, wraps, and hot tubs are forms of hydrotherapy, which is a wonderful tonic for depression and anxiety. Soaking in a tub of steamy hot water or standing under a strong spray of hot water facilitates muscle relaxation and can lift any blue mood.

Psychology Today calls hydrotherapy "the soothing power of soaking." For instance, a hot tub's combination of warmth and pulsing water jets not only quiets a racing mind, but also alleviates body tension. Hot water dilates blood vessels, which improves blood circulation and transports more oxygen to the brain. If you're into bathing, then I recommend adding essential oils, Epsom salts, or herbs to the bath to enhance the therapeutic benefits.

You could also consider trying a brisk, cold shower for a minute or so, which stimulates the body and boosts oxygen use in the cells. One of the healthy habits I do is alternating between hot water and cold water when I shower in the morning and evening. I warm up my body first with hot water, then slowly switch from hot to luke-warm to cool to as cold as I can stand it.

I'm also a personal fan of saunas, since I have a portable far infrared sauna at home, which I've been using for more than eight years. Saunas are a great way to detoxify the body of harm-ful environmental chemicals, fat-soluble toxins, and heavy met-als, and they provide a comfortable and simple way to improve health. (For more information on far infrared sauna technology visit, www.BiblicalHealthInstitute.com.)

Finally, pamper yourself with aromatherapy and music ther-apy. In aromatherapy, essential oils from plants, flowers, and spices are introduced to your skin and pores either by rubbing them in or inhaling their aromas. The use of these essential oils will not miraculously lift your depression, but they will give you an emotional lift. Try rubbing a few drops of myrtle, coriander, hyssop, galbanum, or frankincense onto the palms, then cup your hands over your mouth and nose and inhale. A deep breath will invigorate a wounded spirit.

So will listening to soft and soothing music that promotes relaxation and healing. I know what I like when it comes to music therapy: contemporary praise and worship music. No matter what works for you, you'll find that listening to uplifting "mood" music can heal the body, soul, and spirit.

THE GREAT PHYSICIAN'S RX FOR DEPRESSION AND ANXIETY: CONDITION YOUR BODY WITH EXERCISE AND BODY THERAPIES

- *Make a commitment and an appointment to exercise three times a week or more.*

- *Incorporate five to fifteen minutes of functional fitness into your daily schedule.*

- *Take a brisk walk and see how much better you feel at the end of the day.*

- *Make a conscious effort to practice deep-breathing exercises once a day. Inflate your lungs to full and hold for several seconds before slowly exhaling.*

- *Each Saturday or Sunday, take a day of rest. Dedicate the day to the Lord and do something fun and relaxing that you haven't done in a while. Make your rest day work-free, errand-free, and shop-free. Trust God that He'll do more with His six days than you can do with seven.*

- *Go to sleep earlier, paying close attention to how much sleep you get before midnight. Do your best to get eight hours of sleep nightly.*

- End your next shower by changing the water temperature to cool (or cold) and standing underneath the spray for one minute.

- Once each day, sit outside in a chair and face the sun. Soak up the rays for ten or fifteen minutes but do so before 10 a.m. or after 2 p.m..

- Incorporate essential oils into your daily life.

- Play worship music in your home, in your car, or on your iPod. Focus on God's plan for your life.

Take Action

To learn how to incorporate the principles of conditioning your body with exercise and body therapies into your daily life, please turn to page 74 for the Great Physician's Rx for Depression and Anxiety Battle Plan.

KEY #5

Reduce Toxins in Your Environment

If you were to ever have your blood and urine tested for various chemicals and toxins inside your body because of your depression, the results may startle you: lab technicians would likely uncover dozens of toxins in your bloodstream, including PCBs (polychlorinated biphenyls), dioxins, furans, trace metals, phthalates, VOCs (volatile organic compounds), and chlorine. Scientists refer to this chemical residue as a person's *body burden*, which proves that we are not only what we eat, but we are also what we absorb from the environment.

Although our bodies are designed to eliminate toxins, our bodies have become overloaded because of the chemicals and toxins present in the foods we eat, the air we breathe, and the water we drink. Some toxins are water soluble, meaning they are rapidly passed out of the body and present no harm. Unfortunately, many more toxins are fat soluble, meaning that an overworked elimination system may need months or years before it completely eliminates these toxins from your system. Some of the better-known fat-soluble toxins are dioxins, phthalates, and chlorine.

Chlorine, which is added to municipal water supplies and found in backyard pools, kills bacteria on contact—including beneficial microbes in the gut and on the skin. Remember, when your "second brain" isn't happy, your mood drops like an elevator. The best way to flush fat-soluble toxins out of your bloodstream is by increasing your intake of pure drinking water, which helps eliminate toxins through the kidneys. You must increase the fiber in your diet to eliminate toxins through the bowel, exercise and sweat to eliminate toxins through the lymphatic system, and practice deep breathing to eliminate toxins through the lungs.

Another way to reduce the number of toxins is to consume organic and grass-fed meat and dairy products. Remember: most commercially produced beef and chicken act as chemical magnets for toxins in the environment, so they will not be as healthy as eating organic and grass-fed meats. In addition, consuming organic produce purchased at health food stores, roadside stands, and farmer's markets (only if produce is grown locally and unsprayed) will expose you to less pesticide residues, as compared to conventionally grown fruits and vegetables.

Typical canned tuna is another food to eat minimally, although many popular diets include tuna and tuna salad as a lunchtime or dinner staple. Metallic particles of mercury, lead, and aluminum continue to be found in the fatty tissues of tuna, swordfish, and king mackerel. However, there is now a canned tuna available that is not only low in mercury, but high in omega-3 fatty acids. This tuna can be safely consumed many times per week and contains even more heart-healthy omega-3 fats (such as EPA and DHA) than fatty fish such as salmon and sardines. (For information on low mercury, high omega-3 tuna, visit www.BiblicalHealthInstitute.com and click on the GPRx Resource Guide.)

Housework

You may not have paid much attention to the household cleaners beneath your kitchen sink or stored in bathroom cabinets. These cleaning products usually contain potentially harmful chemicals and solvents that expose people to VOCs (volatile organic compounds), which can cause eye, nose, and throat irritation. Furniture polish, air fresheners, adhesives, and household cleaners are filled with VOCs as well as semivolatile organic chemicals. Synthetic room fresheners and fragranced cleaning products are among the worst offenders, making indoor air unhealthy and provoking skin, eye, and respiratory reactions.

Since stay-at-home moms and preschool children spend 90 percent of their time indoors, according to the American Lung Association, you can see why this should be a concern. In homes where aerosol sprays and air fresheners were used frequently, mothers suffered 25 percent more headaches and 19 percent more depression, and infants under six months of age had 30 percent more ear infections and 22 percent higher incidence of diarrhea, according to a study done at Bristol University in England.[1]

I look to the *Safe Shopper's Bible*, coauthored by my friend David Steinman, for recommendations regarding indoor air quality. First of all, you can quit buying air fresheners, deodorizers, and odor removers. Besides purchasing more indoor houseplants, you should bring home flower sachets and place them in strategic areas around the house. Health food stores also sell fragrance jars and dried botanicals.

What to Drink

I've already touted the healthy benefits of drinking water, but when it comes to reducing toxins in your environment, water is especially important because of its ability to flush out toxins and other metabolic waste from the body. The importance of drinking enough water cannot be overstated: water is a life force involved in nearly every bodily process, from digestion to blood circulation. As Dr. Batmanghelidj said in Key #1, dehydration lowers the level of energy generation in the brain, which results in depression.

The answer to hydration is plain old water—a liquid created by God to be totally compatible with your body. You should be drinking a minimum of eight glasses of water daily, although I think it's better to drink a half-ounce of water per pound of body weight, meaning that if you weigh 150 pounds, you should be drinking seventy-five ounces of water per day.

I don't recommend drinking water straight from the tap, however. Nearly all municipal water is routinely treated with chlorine or chloramine, potent bacteria-killing chemicals that are toxic to all organs and systems of the body. I've installed a whole-house filtration system that removes the chlorine and other impurities out of the water *before* it enters our household pipes. My wife, Nicki, and I can confidently turn on the tap and enjoy the health benefits of chemical-, germ-, and chlorine-free water for drinking, cooking, and bathing. Since our water doesn't have a chemical aftertaste, we're more apt to drink it.

When I'm at the office or out and about, I sip on bottled water all day long. My feelings are that given a choice, you're better off purchasing bottled water from a natural spring source, although filtered tap water (Dasani and Aquafina, for example) would be okay, too. My favorite bottled water brands are Mountain Valley Spring Water, Volvic Natural Spring Water, Trinity Springs Water, and Nariwa Water. All of these bottled waters come from natural springs and have God-given nutrients, purity, and energy. (For more information on my favorite bottled waters, visit www.Biblical HealthInstitute.com, and click on the GPRx Resource Guide.)

THE GREAT PHYSICIAN'S RX FOR DEPRESSION AND ANXIETY: REDUCE TOXINS IN YOUR ENVIRONMENT

- *Eat organic meat from grass-fed sources to lower your exposure to environmental toxins.*

- *When eating canned fish, look for low mercury, high omega-3 sources of tuna.*

- *Drink the recommended eight glasses of water daily—or a half-ounce of water for every pound of body weight.*

- *Use glass containers instead of plastic containers whenever possible.*

- *Improve indoor air quality by opening windows, purchasing houseplants, and buying an air filtration system.*

- *Use natural cleaning products for your home.*

- *Use natural products for skin care, body care, hair care, cosmetics, and toothpaste.*

Take Action

To learn how to incorporate the principles of reducing toxins in your environment, please turn to page 74 for the Great Physician's Rx for Depression and Anxiety Battle Plan.

KEY #6

Avoid Deadly Emotions

At the age of seventeen, on the cusp of adulthood, Angela Roysdon knew something wasn't right. She was never happy—no matter what she did or where she went. Nothing could shake her out of her doldrums.

Her dad had been in the hospital ICU for months, hanging on to life with a set of clogged arteries to his heart. Her mother maintained an exhaustive vigil at her husband's bedside, returning home after dinnertime and retreating straight to bed. Feeling neglected, Angela coped by inviting friends—"good church kids," she said—over to the house to lift her spirits, but she could never step away from the black cloud that followed her everywhere.

"I was in a self-destruct mode," she said. "I didn't eat a whole lot. I had no energy. It was hard to get out of bed."

Her father never recovered and eventually died. Angela fell in with the wrong crowd during her senior year of high school, even though she had grown up in a solid Christian home. I'll let Angela, now in her midtwenties, pick up her story in her own words:

> A year after my father's death, I'll never forget the time when I was lying in bed one night, praying for God to mold me and shape me, when flashbulb memories started to break loose— memories of molestation that happened when I was a little girl.

63

These memories transported me into the throes of deep depression. I tried everything to fill the void—everything except coming back to God. Before I knew it, I was pregnant and marrying a man who would become very abusive to me and our two children. I fell further into the black hole of depression. By my third anniversary, I was living in a safe house, where I was served with divorce papers.

The children and I went to live with my mother, who helped me realize that I needed the Lord. I started attending church regularly and felt myself growing closer to God. Then I would hit a brick wall and struggle. More depression.

I enrolled in a "Change of Heart" class at church, which helped me forgive the seventeen-year-old boy who had done some terrible things to me. Since the molestation, though, I had always struggled with my weight, topping the chart with 320 pounds. I thought about having gastric bypass surgery.

Then in September 2004, I met a man with two children the same ages as my daughter, Hunter, and son, Logan. Jason and I became close and were married in December 2005. Shortly before we were married, we were at a dinner party with some friends and my niece, who is only nine months younger than me, and she asked to have a private conversation with me.

We walked over to a corner of the living room, where she told me about repressed memories about a boy who had molested her—the same boy who had taken advantage of me at a small church in North Carolina. Many of the things I had repressed came to my memory as I listened to my niece tell her story. My mind was screaming, *Oh, God, I've been raped.* Some of the things that were done were gruesome. For instance, my ob-gyn had asked me about scars on my cervix when my daughter was born, but I had no idea where they had come from.

When we left the dinner party, I told Jason about my conversation with my niece. About halfway into it, he said he couldn't take it anymore. "I love you and support you 150 percent, and I will be at your side through all this, but we need to find someone for you to talk to."

That night, more memories came back to my mind. I remember lying on my Sunday school room floor while I was being raped, looking up to the picture of Jesus, silently begging Him to help me. *Please, Jesus, make him stop.*

I received more counseling and prayer for deliverance. I forgave my tormentor again. Some time later, Jordan Rubin came to our church, and I told Jason afterward that I wanted to take the 7 Weeks of Wellness challenge that our church was going through. This 49-day program was based on the Great Physician's prescription for health and wellness.

I started losing weight immediately after starting the program. I felt so much healthier and had more energy. When we got to the sixth week and Key #6, "Avoid Deadly Emotions," I prayed, *God, have I forgiven everyone?*

I kept hearing a voice saying, *No, not everyone.*

Our teacher that evening told us that she had been put on bed rest days before her wedding, which threw her for a loop. She said her mother came by to see her and asked her if she had not forgiven God for something. That's when I felt my breath catch in my throat.

God, am I mad at You? I asked. The Lord brought back memories of the rape and looking up at the picture of Jesus. He spoke to my spirit and said, *I love you, and I have never wanted anything bad for you.*

"God, I am so sorry," I prayed. "I've held this against You." As I wept, I felt a huge weight lift off me. I was no longer depressed, no longer anxious about the future. I felt free and happy for the first time in many, many years.

Dealing with a childhood molestation, a death of a father before high school graduation, a lousy marriage, and life as a single-parent mom—I think we can all nod our heads and say we understand why Angela Roysdon battled depression and unforgiveness in her heart. As much as she had been hurt, Angela put her past in the rearview mirror, expressed her sorrow to the Lord for holding the molestation against Him, and moved forward.

What about you? Are you harboring resentment in your heart, nursing a grudge into overtime, or plotting revenge against those who hurt you? If you're still bottling up emotions such as anger, bitterness, and resentment, these deadly emotions will produce toxins similar to bingeing on a dozen glazed doughnuts. The efficiency of your immune system decreases noticeably for about six hours, and staying angry and bitter about those who have hurt you in the past can alter the chemistry of your brain and your physical body—and make you feel even more depressed. An old proverb states it well: "What you are eating is not nearly as important as what's eating you."

Following the Great Physician's prescription for a healthy lifestyle helped Angela deal with the deadly emotions weighing her down. As for you, please remember that no matter how badly you've been hurt in the past, it's still possible to forgive others. "If you forgive men their trespasses, your heavenly Father will also forgive you," Jesus said. "But if you do not forgive men their trespasses, neither will your Father forgive your trespasses" (Matt. 6:14–15 NKJV).

Give your forgiveness to those who tormented you, hurt you, and made you angry, and then let it go.

℞ THE GREAT PHYSICIAN'S RX FOR DEPRESSION AND ANXIETY: AVOID DEADLY EMOTIONS

- *Don't eat when you're sad, scared, or angry.*

- *Recognize the interaction between deadly emotions and not following a healthy lifestyle.*

- *Trust God when you face circumstances that cause you to worry or become anxious.*

- *Practice forgiveness every day, and forgive those who hurt you.*

Take Action

To learn how to incorporate the principles of avoiding deadly emotions, please turn to page 74 for the Great Physician's Rx for Depression and Anxiety Battle Plan.

KEY #7

Live a Life of Prayer and Purpose

I'll never forget the black cloud that enveloped me when a series of health challenges began when I was nineteen years old. As I described in greater detail in *The Great Physician's Rx for Health and Wellness*, I had just finished my freshman year at Florida State University when I began experiencing nausea, stomach cramps, and horrible digestive problems. The constant diarrhea was the worst—sometimes I had to run to a toilet twenty times a day!

I returned to Florida State for my sophomore year, but I was in no shape to do anything. Each night, 104-degree fever racked my body. My health was so poor that I had to quit the Florida State cheerleading team, say good-bye to my fraternity buddies, and drop out of school. I flew home to Palm Beach Gardens, where I landed in bed and fought fever spikes, vomiting, night sweats, loss of appetite, general feeling of weakness, severe abdominal cramps, and diarrhea—often bloody.

My health deteriorated. I could barely walk. My doctors struggled to find answers until my gastroenterologist finally diagnosed me with Crohn's disease. He informed me that if I didn't get better soon, I would be looking at surgery.

"What kind of surgery?" I asked.

My doctor rattled off words like *resection* and *colectomy* and *ostomy*, and none of those foreign-sounding words sounded good to me. When I asked for explanation, I was told in plain English that my colon would be removed and reattached to an opening the surgeons would make in my abdominal wall. I would then have to wear an "appliance," which was really a bag, to collect my fecal waste.

At the age of nineteen, wearing those crummy bags for the rest of my life sounded like a fate worse than death. Talk about depressing.

In an act of desperation, I boarded a flight for Frankfurt, Germany, and was driven to a small town called Bad Steben, where I received an experimental intravenous drug made from the juices of the Venus flytrap plant. Thousands of miles from home, trapped in a room with a five-foot ceiling, and treated by indifferent nurses who didn't speak English, I felt as though I was imprisoned in my own body. A cloud of despair settled over me. Dr. Helmut Keller, who was treating me, informed my parents that I was clinically depressed.

The experimental treatment didn't work. Another failure, but I really hit bottom when I tried to board my flight back to the United States. No one at the ticket counter spoke English. They had no record of me in the computer. My credit card was declined when I attempted to purchase a new ticket.

Out of options, out of hope, I felt sorry for myself. My body was reeling from chronic bowel problems, a painful urinary tract infection, and a case of double conjunctivitis—pinkeye. Standing at the ticket counter, I closed my eyes and prayed, "Lord, I can't do a single thing. I'm putting my life in your hands. Please help me get home." Within minutes, my ticket was found in the computer. I can't describe how relieved I felt to get back to the United States.

I wasn't out of the woods, but I clung to Jeremiah 29:11: "I know the plans I have for you . . . plans to prosper you and not to harm you, plans to give you hope and a future" (NIV). Eventually God led me to the very keys that I write about in this book, and He healed me.

Right about now, you may not think God has any sort of plan for you, but He does. The Lord is not done with you yet. If you have a relationship with Him, you can talk to God anytime, anywhere, for any reason. He is always there to listen, and He always has our best interests at heart, because we are His children. When my health spun out of control, I didn't have much else to hang on to but the Lord. In my darkest hour, I spoke with Him constantly.

Prayer is how we talk to God. There is no greater source of power than talking to the One who made us. Prayer is not a formality. Prayer is not about religion. Prayer is about a relationship—the hotline to heaven. At times I felt as if I heard God's voice in reply, while on other occasions He directed me to Scriptures that seemed particularly relevant to my dire situation. What God was teaching me was to listen to Him. Jesus said, "My sheep listen to my voice" (John 10:27 NIV), and I count myself among His flock.

Another Scripture seemed particularly apt for my situation: "Blessed is the man who listens to me, watching daily at my doors, waiting at my doorway. For whoever finds me finds life and receives favor from the LORD" (Prov. 8:34–35 NIV). Sometimes when I prayed, the Lord put things on my heart that I hadn't even thought about before I started. (Don't forget that prayer is actually a two-way communication with God.) Sometimes He didn't answer my prayers in the way I expected Him to, but He transformed my heart to align with His.

In living a healthy, purpose-filled life, prayer is the most powerful tool that we possess. Prayer connects the entire person—body, mind, and spirit—to God. Through prayer, God takes away our guilt, shame, bitterness, and anger and gives us a brand-new heart and a brand-new start. We can eat organic whole foods, supplement our diet with whole food supplements, practice advanced hygiene, reduce toxins, and exercise like crazy, but if the spirit is not where it needs to be with God, then we will never be completely healthy. Talking to our Maker through prayer is the foundation for conquering depression and anxiety, and it makes us whole. After all, God's love and grace are our greatest foods for mind, body, and spirit.

The seventh key to unlocking your health potential is living a life of prayer and purpose. Prayer will confirm your purpose, and it will give you the perseverance to complete it. Seal all that you do with the power of prayer, and watch your life become more than you ever thought possible.

START A SMALL GROUP

It's difficult to deal with depression and anxiety alone. If you have friends or family members who are struggling, ask them to join you in following the Great Physician's Rx 7 Weeks of Wellness small group program. To learn about joining an existing group in your area or leading a small group in your church, please visit www.BiblicalHealthInstitute.com.

℞ THE GREAT PHYSICIAN'S RX FOR DEPRESSION AND ANXIETY: LIVE A LIFE OF PRAYER AND PURPOSE

- *Pray continually.*

- *Confess God's promises upon waking and before you retire.*

- *Find God's purpose for your life and live it.*

- *Be an agent of change in your life by adopting the 7 Keys into your life.*

Take Action

To learn how to incorporate the principles of living a life of prayer and purpose into your daily life, please turn to page 74 for the Great Physician's Rx for Depression and Anxiety Battle Plan.

THE GREAT PHYSICIAN'S RX FOR DEPRESSION AND ANXIETY BATTLE PLAN

DAY 1

Upon Waking

Prayer: thank God because this is the day that the Lord has made. Rejoice and be glad in it. Thank Him for the breath in your lungs and the life in your body. Ask the Lord to heal your body and mind and use your experience to benefit the lives of others. Read Matthew 6:9–13 out loud.

Purpose: ask the Lord to give you an opportunity to add significance to someone's life today. Watch for that opportunity. Ask God to use you this day for His intended purpose.

Advanced hygiene: for hands and nails, jab fingers into semisoft soap four or five times, and lather hands with soap for fifteen seconds, rubbing soap over cuticles and rinsing under water as warm as you can stand. Take another swab of semisoft soap into your hands and wash your face. Next, fill basin or sink with water as warm as you can stand, and add one to three tablespoons of table salt and one to three eyedroppers of iodine-based mineral solution. Dunk your face into the water and open your eyes, blinking repeatedly underwater. Keep your eyes open underwater for three seconds. After cleaning your eyes, put your face back in the water, and close your mouth while blowing bubbles out of your nose. Come up from the water, and immerse your face in the water once again, gently taking water into your nostrils and expelling bubbles. Come up from the water, and blow your nose into facial tissue. To cleanse the ears, use hydrogen peroxide and mineral-based ear drops, putting two or three drops into each ear and letting it

74

stand for sixty seconds. Tilt your head to expel the drops. For the teeth, apply two or three drops of essential oil–based tooth drops to the toothbrush. This can be used to brush your teeth or added to existing toothpaste. After brushing your teeth, brush your tongue for fifteen seconds. (For recommended advanced hygiene products, visit www.Biblical HealthInstitute.com and click on the Resource Guide.)

Reduce toxins: open your windows for one hour today. Use natural soap and natural skin and body care products (shower gel, body creams, etc.). Use natural facial care products. Use natural toothpaste. Use natural hair care products such as shampoo, conditioner, gel, mousse, and hairspray. (For recommended products, visit www.BiblicalHealth Institute.com and click on the Resource Guide.)

Supplements: take one serving of a whole food fiber powder with flaxseed mixed in twelve to sixteen ounces of water, and swallow three capsules of a whole food probiotic formula with soil-based organisms. (For recommended products, visit www.BiblicalHealthInstitute.com and click on the Resource Guide.)

Body therapy: get twenty minutes of direct sunlight sometime during the day, but be careful between the hours of 10 a.m. and 2 p.m.

Exercise: perform functional fitness exercises for five to fifteen minutes or spend five to fifteen minutes on a mini-trampoline. Finish with five to ten minutes of deep-breathing exercises. (One to three rounds of the exercises can be found at www.BiblicalHealthInstitute.com.)

Emotional health: whenever you face a circumstance, such as your health challenge, that causes you to worry, repeat the following: "Lord, I trust You. I cast my cares upon You, and I believe that You're going to take care of [insert your current situation] and cause me to be healthy and in sound mind and body." Confess that throughout the day whenever you think about your health challenge.

Breakfast

Make a smoothie in a blender with the following ingredients:

1 cup plain yogurt or kefir (sheep's milk is best)

1 tablespoon organic flaxseed oil

1 tablespoon organic raw honey

1 cup of organic fruit (berries, banana, peaches, pineapple, etc.)

2 tablespoons goat's milk protein powder (for recommended products, visit www.BiblicalHealthInstitute.com and click on the Resource Guide)

dash of vanilla extract (optional)

Supplements: take two whole food multivitamin caplets and one caplet of an adaptogenic herbal formula with B vitamins (for recommended products, visit www.BiblicalHealthInstitute.com and click on the Resource Guide).

Lunch

Before eating, drink eight ounces of water.

During lunch, drink eight ounces of water or hot tea with honey.

large green salad with mixed greens, avocado, carrots, tomato, red cabbage, red onion, red pepper, and sprouts with three hard-boiled omega-3 eggs

salad dressing: mix extra virgin olive oil, apple cider vinegar or lemon juice, minced fresh garlic, naturally brewed soy sauce, Celtic sea salt, herbs, and spices together; or, mix one tablespoon of extra virgin olive oil with one tablespoon of a healthy store-bought dressing

one apple with skin

Supplements: take two whole food multivitamin caplets and one caplet of an adaptogenic herbal formula with B vitamins.

Dinner

Before eating, drink eight ounces of water.

During dinner, drink hot tea with honey (for recommended brands, visit www.BiblicalHealthInstitute.com and click on the Resource Guide).

baked, poached, or grilled wild-caught salmon

steamed broccoli

large green salad with mixed greens, avocado, carrots, tomato, red cabbage, red onion, red pepper, and sprouts

salad dressing: mix extra virgin olive oil, apple cider vinegar or lemon juice, minced fresh garlic, naturally brewed soy sauce, Celtic sea salt, herbs, and spices together; or, mix one tablespoon of extra virgin olive oil with one tablespoon of a healthy store-bought dressing

Supplements: take two whole food multivitamin caplets, one caplet of an adaptogenic herbal formula with B vitamins, and one to three teaspoons or three to nine capsules of a high omega-3 cod liver oil complex (for recommended products, visit www.BiblicalHealthInstitute.com and click on the Resource Guide).

Snacks

Drink eight to twelve ounces of water, or hot or iced fresh-brewed tea with honey.

one serving of healthy cacao (chocolate) snack (for recommended products, visit www.BiblicalHealthInstitute.com and click on the Resource Guide)

one whole food nutrition bar with beta-glucans from soluble oat fiber (for recommended products, visit www.BiblicalHealthInstitute.com and click on the Resource Guide)

Before Bed

Exercise: go for a walk outdoors or participate in a favorite sport or recreational activity.

Supplements: take one serving of a whole food fiber powder with flaxseed mixed in twelve to sixteen ounces of water, and swallow three capsules of a whole food probiotic formula with soil-based organisms.

Body therapy: take a warm bath for fifteen minutes with eight drops of biblical essential oils added.

Advanced hygiene: repeat the advanced hygiene instructions from the morning of Day 1.

Emotional health: ask the Lord to bring to your mind someone you need to forgive. Take a sheet of paper and write the person's name at the top. Try to remember each specific action that person did against you that brought you pain. Write down the following: "I forgive [insert person's name] for [insert the action he or she did against you]." After you fill the paper, tear it up or burn it, and ask God to give you the strength to truly forgive that person.

Purpose: ask yourself these questions: "Did I live a life of purpose today?" "What did I do to add value to someone else's life today?" Commit to living a day of purpose tomorrow.

Prayer: thank God for this day, asking Him to give you a restoring night's rest and a fresh start tomorrow. Thank Him for His steadfast love that never ceases and His mercies that are new every morning. Read Romans 8:35, 37–39 aloud.

Sleep: go to bed by 10:30 p.m.

Day 2

Upon Waking

Prayer: thank God because this is the day that the Lord has made. Rejoice and be glad in it. Thank Him for the breath in your lungs and the life in your body. Ask the Lord to heal your body and mind and use your experience to benefit the lives of others. Read Psalm 91 aloud.

Purpose: ask the Lord to give you an opportunity to add significance to someone's life today. Watch for that opportunity. Ask God to use you this day for His intended purpose.

Advanced hygiene: follow the advanced hygiene recommendations from the morning of Day 1.

Reduce toxins: follow the recommendations to reduce toxins from the morning of Day 1.

Supplements: take one serving of a whole food fiber powder with flaxseed mixed in twelve to sixteen ounces of water, and swallow three capsules of a whole food probiotic formula with soil-based organisms.

Body therapy: take a hot and cold shower. After a normal shower, alternate sixty seconds of water as hot as you can stand it, followed by sixty seconds of water as cold as you can stand it. Repeat this cycle four times for a total of eight minutes, finishing with cold.

Exercise: perform functional fitness exercises for five to fifteen minutes or spend five to fifteen minutes on a mini-trampoline. Finish with five to ten minutes of deep-breathing exercises. (One to three rounds of the exercises can be found at www.BiblicalHealthInstitute.com.)

Emotional health: follow the emotional health recommendations from the morning of Day 1.

Breakfast

two or three omega-3 eggs any style, cooked in one tablespoon of extra virgin coconut oil (for recommended products, visit www.Biblical HealthInstitute.com and click on the Resource Guide)

stir-fried onions, mushrooms, and peppers

one slice of sprouted or yeast-free whole grain bread with almond butter and honey

Supplements: take two whole food multivitamin caplets and one caplet of an adaptogenic herbal formula with B-vitamins.

Lunch

Before eating, drink eight ounces of water.

During lunch, drink eight ounces of water or hot tea with honey.

large green salad with mixed greens, avocado, carrots, tomato, red cabbage, red onions, red pepper, and sprouts with two ounces of low mercury, high omega-3 tuna (for recommended products, visit www.BiblicalHealthInstitute.com and click on the Resource Guide)

salad dressing, mix extra virgin olive oil, apple cider vinegar or lemon juice, minced fresh garlic, naturally brewed soy sauce, Celtic sea salt, herbs, and spices together; or, mix one tablespoon of extra virgin olive oil with one tablespoon of a healthy store-bought dressing organic grapes

Supplements: take two whole food multivitamin caplets and one caplet of an adaptogenic herbal formula with B-vitamins.

Dinner

Before eating, drink eight ounces of water.

During dinner, drink hot tea with honey.

roasted organic chicken

cooked vegetables (carrots, onions, peas, etc.)

large green salad with mixed greens, avocado, carrots, tomato, red cabbage, red onion, red pepper, and sprouts

salad dressing: mix extra virgin olive oil, apple cider vinegar or lemon juice, minced fresh garlic, naturally brewed soy sauce, Celtic sea salt, herbs, and spices together; or, mix one tablespoon of extra virgin olive oil with one tablespoon of a healthy store-bought dressing

Supplements: take two whole food multivitamin caplets, one caplet of an adaptogenic herbal formula with B vitamins, and one to three teaspoons or three to nine capsules of a high omega-3 cod liver oil complex.

Snacks

Drink eight to twelve ounces of water, or hot or iced fresh-brewed tea with honey.

one serving of a healthy cacao (chocolate) snack

one whole food nutrition bar with beta-glucans from soluble oat fiber

Before Bed

Exercise: go for a walk outdoors or participate in a favorite sport or recreational activity.

Supplements: take one serving of a whole food fiber powder with flaxseed mixed in twelve to sixteen ounces of water, and swallow three capsules of a whole food probiotic formula with soil-based organisms. (For recommended products, visit www.BiblicalHealthInstitute.com and click on the Resource Guide.)

Advanced hygiene: repeat the advanced hygiene instructions from the morning of Day 1.

Emotional health: repeat the emotional health recommendations from Day 1.

Purpose: ask yourself these questions: "Did I live a life of purpose today?" "What did I do to add value to someone else's life today?" Commit to living a day of purpose tomorrow.

Prayer: thank God for this day, asking Him to give you a restoring night's rest and a fresh start tomorrow. Thank Him for His steadfast love that never ceases and His mercies that are new every morning. Read 1 Corinthians 13:4–8 aloud.

Body therapy: spend ten minutes listening to soothing music before you retire.

Sleep: go to bed by 10:30 p.m.

DAY 3

Upon Waking

Prayer: thank God because this is the day that the Lord has made. Rejoice and be glad in it. Thank Him for the breath in your lungs and the life in your body. Ask the Lord to heal your body and mind and use your experience to benefit the lives of others. Read Ephesians 6:13–18 aloud.

Purpose: ask the Lord to give you an opportunity to add significance to someone's life today. Watch for that opportunity. Ask God to use you this day for His intended purpose.

Advanced hygiene: follow the advanced hygiene recommendations from the morning of Day 1.

Reduce toxins: follow the recommendations to reduce toxins from the morning of Day 1.

Supplements: take one serving of a whole food fiber powder with flaxseed mixed in twelve to sixteen ounces of water, and swallow three capsules of a whole food probiotic formula with soil-based organisms.

Body therapy: get twenty minutes of direct sunlight sometime during the day, but be careful between the hours of 10 a.m. and 2 p.m.

Exercise: perform functional fitness exercises for five to fifteen minutes or spend five to fifteen minutes on a mini trampoline. Finish with five to ten minutes of deep-breathing exercises. (One to three rounds of the exercises can be found at www.BiblicalHealthInstitute.com.)

Emotional health: follow the emotional health recommendations from Day 1.

Breakfast

four to eight ounces of organic whole milk yogurt or cottage cheese with fruit (pineapple, peaches, or berries), honey, and a dash of vanilla extract

handful of raw almonds

one cup of hot tea with honey

Supplements: take two whole food multivitamin caplets and one caplet of an adaptogenic herbal formula with B vitamins.

Lunch

Before eating, drink eight ounces of water.

During lunch, drink eight ounces of water or hot tea with honey.

large green salad with mixed greens, avocado, carrots, tomato, red cabbage, red onion, red pepper, and sprouts with three hard-boiled omega-3 eggs

salad dressing: mix extra virgin olive oil, apple cider vinegar or lemon juice, minced fresh garlic, naturally brewed soy sauce, Celtic sea salt, herbs, and spices together; or, mix one tablespoon of extra virgin olive oil with one tablespoon of a healthy store-bought dressing

one piece of fruit in season

Supplements: take two whole food multivitamin caplets and one caplet of an adaptogenic herbal formula with B vitamins.

Dinner

Before eating, drink eight ounces of water.

During dinner, drink hot tea with honey.

red meat steak (beef, buffalo, or venison)

steamed broccoli

baked sweet potato with butter

large green salad with mixed greens, avocado, carrots, tomato, red cabbage, red onion, red pepper, and sprouts

salad dressing: mix extra virgin olive oil, apple cider vinegar or lemon juice, minced fresh garlic, naturally brewed soy sauce, Celtic sea salt, herbs, and spices together; or, mix one tablespoon of extra virgin olive oil with one tablespoon of a healthy store-bought dressing

Supplements: take two whole food multivitamin caplets, one caplet of an adaptogenic herbal formula with B vitamins, and one to three teaspoons or three to nine capsules of a high omega-3 cod liver oil complex.

Snacks

Drink eight to twelve ounces of water, or hot or iced fresh-brewed tea with honey.

one serving of healthy cacao (chocolate) snack

one berry antioxidant whole food nutrition bar with beta-glucans from soluble oat fiber

Before Bed

Exercise: go for a walk outdoors or participate in a favorite sport or recreational activity.

Supplements: take one serving of a whole food fiber powder with flaxseed mixed in twelve to sixteen ounces of water, and swallow three capsules of a whole food probiotic formula with soil-based organisms.

Body therapy: take a warm bath for fifteen minutes with eight drops of biblical essential oils added.

Advanced hygiene: follow the advanced hygiene instructions from the morning of Day 1.

Emotional health: follow the forgiveness recommendations from the evening of Day 1.

Purpose: ask yourself these questions: "Did I live a life of purpose today?" "What did I do to add value to someone else's life today?" Commit to living a day of purpose tomorrow.

Prayer: thank God for this day, asking Him to give you a restoring night's rest and a fresh start tomorrow. Thank Him for His steadfast love that never ceases and His mercies that are new every morning. Read Philippians 4:4–8, 11–13,19 aloud.

Sleep: go to bed by 10:30 p.m.

DAY 4

Upon Waking

Prayer: thank God because this is the day that the Lord has made. Rejoice and be glad in it. Thank Him for the breath in your lungs and the life in your body. Read Matthew 6:9–13 aloud.

Purpose: ask the Lord to give you an opportunity to add significance to someone's life today. Watch for that opportunity. Ask God to use you this day for His intended purpose.

Advanced hygiene: follow the advanced hygiene recommendations from Day 1.

Reduce toxins: follow the recommendations for reducing toxins from Day 1.

Supplements: take one serving of a whole food fiber powder with flaxseed mixed in twelve to sixteen ounces of water, and swallow three capsules of a whole food probiotic formula with soil-based organisms.

Exercise: perform functional fitness exercises for five to fifteen minutes or spend five to fifteen minutes on a mini-trampoline. Finish with five to ten minutes of deep-breathing exercises. (One to three rounds of the exercises can be found at www.BiblicalHealthInstitute.com.)

Body therapy: take a hot and cold shower. After a normal shower, alternate sixty seconds of water as hot as you can stand it, followed by sixty seconds of water as cold as you can stand it. Repeat the cycle four times for a total of eight minutes, finishing with cold.

Emotional health: follow the emotional health recommendations from the morning of Day 1.

Breakfast

three soft-boiled or poached omega-3 eggs

four ounces of sprouted whole grain cereal with two ounces of whole milk yogurt (for recommended products, visit www.BiblicalHealth Institute.com and click on the Resource Guide)

one cup of hot tea with honey

Supplements: take two whole food multivitamin caplets and one caplet of an adaptogenic herbal formula with B-vitamins.

Lunch

Before eating, drink eight ounces of water.

During lunch, drink eight ounces of water or hot tea with honey.

large green salad with mixed greens, avocado, carrots, tomato, red cabbage, red onion, red pepper, and sprouts with three ounces of low mercury, high omega-3 tuna

salad dressing: mix extra virgin olive oil, apple cider vinegar or lemon juice, minced fresh garlic, naturally brewed soy sauce, Celtic sea salt, herbs, and spices together; or, mix one tablespoon of extra virgin olive oil with one tablespoon of a healthy store-bought dressing

one bunch of grapes with seeds

Supplements: take two whole food multivitamin caplets and one caplet of an adaptogenic herbal formula with B vitamins.

Dinner

Before eating, drink eight ounces of water.

During dinner, drink hot tea with honey.

grilled chicken breast

steamed veggies

small portion of cooked non-gluten whole grain (quinoa, amaranth, millet, or buckwheat) cooked with one tablespoon of extra virgin coconut oil

large green salad with mixed greens, avocado, carrots, tomato, red cabbage, red onions red pepper, and sprouts

salad dressing: mix extra virgin olive oil, apple cider vinegar or lemon juice, minced fresh garlic, naturally brewed soy sauce, Celtic sea salt, herbs, and spices together; or, mix one tablespoon of extra virgin olive oil with one tablespoon of a healthy store-bought dressing

Supplements: take two whole food multivitamin caplets, one caplet of an adaptogenic herbal formula with B vitamins, and one to three teaspoons or three to nine capsules of a high omega-3 cod liver oil complex.

Snacks

Drink eight to twelve ounces of water, or hot or iced fresh-brewed tea with honey.

one serving of healthy cacao (chocolate) snack

one berry antioxidant whole food nutrition bar with beta glucans from soluble oat fiber

Before Bed

Drink eight to twelve ounces of water or hot tea with honey.

Exercise: go for a walk outdoors or participate in a favorite sport or recreational activity.

Supplements: take one serving of a whole food fiber powder with flaxseed mixed in twelve to sixteen ounces of water, and swallow three capsules of a whole food probiotic formula with soil-based organisms.

Advanced hygiene: follow the advanced hygiene recommendations from the morning of Day 1.

Emotional health: follow the forgiveness recommendations from the evening of Day 1.

Purpose: ask yourself these questions: "Did I live a life of purpose today?" "What did I do to add value to someone else's life today?" Commit to living a day of purpose tomorrow.

Prayer: thank God for this day, asking Him to give you a restoring night's rest and a fresh start tomorrow. Thank Him for His steadfast love that never ceases and His mercies that are new every morning. Read Romans 8:35, 37–39 aloud.

Body therapy: spend ten minutes listening to soothing music before you retire.

Sleep: go to bed by 10:30 p.m.

Day 5 (Partial Fast Day)

Upon Waking

Prayer: thank God because this is the day that the Lord has made. Rejoice and be glad in it. Thank Him for the breath in your lungs and the life in your body. Read Isaiah 58:6–9 aloud.

Purpose: ask the Lord to give you an opportunity to add significance to someone's life today. Watch for that opportunity. Ask God to use you this day for His intended purpose.

Advanced hygiene: follow the advanced hygiene recommendations from Day 1.

Reduce toxins: follow the recommendations for reducing toxins from Day 1.

Supplements: take one serving of a whole food fiber powder with flaxseed mixed in twelve to sixteen ounces of water, and swallow three capsules of a whole food probiotic formula with soil-based organisms.

Exercise: perform functional fitness exercises for five to fifteen minutes or spend five to fifteen minutes on a mini trampoline. Finish with five to ten minutes of deep-breathing exercises.

Body therapy: get twenty minutes of direct sunlight sometime during the day, but be careful between the hours of 10 a.m. to 2 p.m.

Emotional health: follow the emotional health recommendations from the morning of Day 1.

Breakfast

Drink eight to twelve ounces of water.

no food (partial fast day)

Supplements: none (partial fast day)

Lunch

no food (partial fast day)

Supplements: none (partial fast day)

Dinner

Before eating, drink eight ounces of water.

During dinner, drink hot tea with honey.

chicken soup (visit www.GreatPhysiciansRx.com for the recipe)

cultured vegetables (for recommended products, visit www.Biblical HealthInstitute.com and click on the Resource Guide)

large green salad with mixed greens, avocado, carrots, tomato, red cabbage, red onion, red pepper, and sprouts

salad dressing: mix extra virgin olive oil, apple cider vinegar or lemon juice, minced fresh garlic, naturally brewed soy sauce, Celtic sea salt, herbs, and spices together; or, mix one tablespoon of extra virgin olive oil with one tablespoon of a healthy store-bought dressing

Supplements: take two whole food multivitamin caplets, one caplet of an adaptogenic herbal formula with B vitamins, and one to three teaspoons or three to nine capsules of a high omega-3 cod liver oil complex.

Snacks

Drink eight ounces of water.

no food (partial fast day)

Before Bed

Drink eight to twelve ounces of water or hot tea with honey.

Exercise: go for a walk outdoors or participate in a favorite sport or recreational activity.

Supplements: take one serving of a whole food fiber powder with flaxseed mixed in twelve to sixteen ounces of water and swallow three capsules of a whole food probiotic formula with soil-based organisms.

Advanced hygiene: follow the advanced hygiene recommendations from the morning of Day 1.

Emotional health: follow the forgiveness recommendations from the evening of Day 1.

Body therapy: take a warm bath for fifteen minutes with eight drops of biblical essential oils added.

Purpose: ask yourself these questions: "Did I live a life of purpose today?" "What did I do to add value to someone else's life today?" Commit to living a day of purpose tomorrow.

Prayer: thank God for this day, asking Him to give you a restoring night's rest and a fresh start tomorrow. Thank Him for His steadfast love that never ceases and His mercies that are new every morning. Read Isaiah 58:6–9 aloud.

Sleep: go to bed by 10:30 p.m.

DAY 6 (REST DAY)

Upon Waking

Prayer: thank God because this is the day that the Lord has made. Rejoice and be glad in it. Thank Him for the breath in your lungs and the life in your body. Read Psalm 23 aloud.

Purpose: ask the Lord to give you an opportunity to add significance to someone's life today. Watch for that opportunity. Ask God to use you this day for His intended purpose.

Advanced hygiene: follow the advanced hygiene recommendations from Day 1.

Reduce toxins: follow the recommendations for reducing toxins from Day 1.

Supplements: take one serving of a whole food fiber powder with flaxseed mixed in twelve to sixteen ounces of water, and swallow three capsules of a whole food probiotic formula with soil-based organisms. (For recommended products, visit www.BiblicalHealthInstitute.com and click on the Resource Guide.)

Exercise: no formal exercise since it's a rest day.

Body therapies: none since it's a rest day.

Emotional health: follow the emotional health recommendations from the morning of Day 1.

Breakfast

two or three omega-3 eggs cooked any style in one tablespoon of extra virgin coconut oil

one grapefruit or orange

handful of almonds

Supplements: take two whole food multivitamin caplets and one caplet of an adaptogenic herbal formula with B vitamins.

Lunch

Before eating, drink eight ounces of water.

During lunch, drink eight ounces of water or hot tea with honey.

large green salad with mixed greens, avocado, carrots, tomato, red cabbage, red onion, red pepper, and sprouts with two ounces of low mercury, high omega-3 tuna

salad dressing: mix extra virgin olive oil, apple cider vinegar or lemon juice, minced fresh garlic, naturally brewed soy sauce, Celtic sea salt, herbs, and spices together; or, mix one tablespoon of extra virgin olive oil with one tablespoon of a healthy store-bought dressing

one organic apple with the skin

Supplements: take two whole food multivitamin caplets and one caplet of an adaptogenic herbal formula with B-vitamins. (For recommended products, visit www.BiblicalHealthInstitute.com and click on the Resource Guide).

Dinner

Before eating, drink eight ounces of water.

During dinner, drink hot tea with honey.

roasted organic chicken

cooked vegetables (carrots, onions, peas, etc.)

large green salad with mixed greens, avocado, carrots, tomato, red cabbage, red onion, red pepper, and sprouts

salad dressing: mix extra virgin olive oil, apple cider vinegar or lemon juice, minced fresh garlic, naturally brewed soy sauce, Celtic sea salt, herbs, and spices together; or, mix one tablespoon of extra virgin olive oil with one tablespoon of a healthy store-bought dressing

Supplements: take two whole food multivitamin caplets, one caplet of an adaptogenic herbal formula with B vitamins, and one to three teaspoons or three to nine capsules of a high omega-3 cod liver oil complex.

Snacks

Drink eight to twelve ounces of water, or hot or iced fresh-brewed tea with honey.

one serving of healthy cacao (chocolate) snack

one berry antioxidant whole food nutrition bar with beta-glucans from soluble oat fiber

Before Bed

Drink eight to twelve ounces of water or hot tea with honey.

Exercise: go for a walk outdoors or participate in a favorite sport or recreational activity.

Supplements: take one serving of a whole food fiber powder with flaxseed mixed in twelve to sixteen ounces of water, and swallow three capsules of a whole food probiotic formula with soil-based organisms.

Advanced hygiene: follow the advanced hygiene recommendations from the morning of Day 1.

Emotional health: follow the forgiveness recommendations from the evening of Day 1.

Purpose: ask yourself these questions: "Did I live a life of purpose today?" "What did I do to add value to someone else's life today?" Commit to living a day of purpose tomorrow.

Prayer: thank God for this day, asking Him to give you a restoring night's rest and a fresh start tomorrow. Thank Him for His steadfast love that never ceases and His mercies that are new every morning. Read Psalm 23 aloud.

Body therapy: spend ten minutes listening to soothing music before you retire.

Sleep: go to bed by 10:30 p.m.

Day 7

Upon Waking

Prayer: thank God because this is the day that the Lord has made. Rejoice and be glad in it. Thank Him for the breath in your lungs and the life in your body. Read Psalm 91 aloud.

Purpose: ask the Lord to give you an opportunity to add significance to someone's life today. Watch for that opportunity. Ask God to use you this day for His intended purpose.

Advanced hygiene: follow the advanced hygiene recommendations from Day 1.

Reduce toxins: follow the recommendations for reducing toxins from Day 1.

Supplements: take one serving of a whole food fiber powder with flaxseed mixed in twelve to sixteen ounces of water, and swallow three capsules of a whole food probiotic formula with soil-based organisms.

Exercise: perform functional fitness exercises for five to fifteen minutes or spend five to fifteen minutes on a mini-trampoline. Finish with five to ten minutes of deep-breathing exercises.

Body therapy: get twenty minutes of direct sunlight sometime during the day, but be careful between the hours of 10 a.m. and 2 p.m.

Emotional health: follow the emotional health recommendations from the morning of Day 1.

Breakfast

Make a smoothie in a blender with the following ingredients:

1 cup plain yogurt or kefir (sheep's milk is best)

1 tablespoon organic flaxseed oil

1 tablespoon organic raw honey

1 cup of organic fruit (berries, banana, peaches, pineapple, etc.)

2 tablespoons goat's milk protein powder

dash of vanilla extract (optional)

Supplements: take two whole food multivitamin caplets and one caplet of an adaptogenic herbal formula with B-vitamins.

Lunch

Before eating, drink eight ounces of water.

During lunch, drink eight ounces of water or hot tea with honey.

large green salad with mixed greens, avocado, carrots, tomato, red cabbage, red onion, red pepper, and sprouts with three ounces of cold, poached, or canned wild-caught salmon

salad dressing: mix extra virgin olive oil, apple cider vinegar or lemon juice, minced fresh garlic, naturally brewed soy sauce, Celtic sea salt, herbs, and spices together; or, mix one tablespoon of extra virgin olive oil with one tablespoon of a healthy store-bought dressing

one piece of fruit in season

Supplements: take two whole food multivitamin caplets and one caplet of an adaptogenic herbal formula with B vitamins.

Dinner

Before eating, drink eight ounces of water.

During dinner, drink hot tea with honey.

baked or grilled fish of your choice

steamed broccoli

baked sweet potato with butter

large green salad with mixed greens, avocado, carrots, tomato, red cabbage, red onion, red pepper, and sprouts

salad dressing: mix extra virgin olive oil, apple cider vinegar or lemon juice, minced fresh garlic, naturally brewed soy sauce, Celtic sea salt, herbs, and spices together; or, mix one tablespoon of extra virgin olive oil with one tablespoon of a healthy store-bought dressing

Supplements: take two whole food multivitamin caplets, one caplet of an adaptogenic herbal formula with B-vitamins, and one to three teaspoons or three to nine capsules of a high omega-3 cod liver oil complex.

Snacks

Drink eight to twelve ounces of water, or hot or iced fresh-brewed tea with honey.

one serving of healthy cacao (chocolate) snack

one berry antioxidant whole food nutrition bar with beta-glucans from soluble oat fiber

Before Bed

Drink eight to twelve ounces of water or hot tea with honey.

Exercise: go for a walk outdoors or participate in a favorite sport or recreational activity.

Supplements: take one serving of a whole food fiber powder with flaxseed mixed in twelve to sixteen ounces of water and swallow three capsules of a whole food probiotic formula with soil-based organisms.

Advanced hygiene: follow the advanced hygiene recommendations from the morning of Day 1.

Emotional health: follow the forgiveness recommendations from the evening of Day 1.

Body therapy: take a warm bath for fifteen minutes with eight drops of biblical essential oils added.

Purpose: ask yourself these questions: "Did I live a life of purpose today?" "What did I do to add value to someone else's life today?" Commit to living a day of purpose tomorrow.

Prayer: thank God for this day, asking Him to give you a restoring night's rest and a fresh start tomorrow. Thank Him for His steadfast love that never ceases and His mercies that are new every morning. Read 1 Corinthians 13:4-8 aloud.

Sleep: go to bed by 10:30 p.m.

DAY 8 AND BEYOND

If you're feeling better, you can repeat the Great Physician's Rx for Depression and Anxiety Battle Plan as many times as you'd like. For detailed step-by-step suggestions and meal and lifestyle plans, visit www.GreatPhysiciansRx.com and join the 40 Day Health Experience for continued good health. Or, you may be interested in the Lifetime of Wellness plan if you want to maintain your newfound level of health. These online programs will provide you with customized daily meal and exercise plans and provide you with the tools to track your progress.

If you've experienced positive results from *The Great Physician's Rx for Depression and Anxiety,* I encourage you to reach out to someone you know and recommend this book and Battle Plan to them. You can learn how to lead a small group at your church or home by visiting www.BiblicalHealthInstitute.com.

Remember: you don't have to be a doctor or a health expert to help transform the life of someone you care about—you just have to be willing.

Allow me to offer this prayer of blessing from Numbers 6:24–27 NKJV to you:

The LORD bless you and keep you;
The LORD make His face shine upon you,
And be gracious to you;
The LORD lift up His countenance upon you,
And give you peace.

NEED RECIPES?

For a detailed list of over two hundred healthy and delicious recipes contained in the Great Physician's Rx eating plan, please visit www.BiblicalHealthInstitute.com.

NOTES

Introduction

1. Aaron Smith, "The Antidepressants to Watch in '06," CNNMoney.com, http://money.cnn.com/2006/01/04/news/companies/antidepressants/index.htm (accessed March 16, 2007).

2. James F. Balch, M.D., and Mark Stengler, N.D., *Prescription for Natural Cures* (Hoboken, NJ: John Wiley & Sons, Inc., 2004), 182.

3. "Depression," University of Maryland Medical Center, http://www.umm.edu/altmed/ConsConditions/Depressioncc.html (accessed March 16, 2007).

4. Phyllis A. Balch, C.N.C., *Prescription for Nutritional Healing* (Wayne, NJ: Avery Publishing, 2000), 315.

5. Miranda Hitti, "Depression May Be in the Genes," WedMD, http://www.webmd.com/news/20060926/depression-may-be-in-genes, (accessed September 26, 2006).

6. Ellen W. Freeman, Ph.D., "Understanding PMS," University of Pennsylvania Health System, http://www.obgyn.upenn.edu/mudd/PMSarticle.html (accessed March 16, 2007).

7. Laurie Barclay, "'Baby Blues' Don't Have to Grow to Full-Blown Depression," WebMD, http://www.webmd.com/content/article/31/1728_77400.htm (accessed March 16, 2007).

8. Dani Veracity, "Achieve Optimum Mental Health by Supplementing Deficient Brain Chemicals Instead of Resorting to Dangerous Antidepressant Drugs," Newstarget.com, http://www.newstarget.com/019327.html (accessed March 16, 2007).

9. Franklin Sanders, "The Mood Cure," The Moneychanger, http://www.the-moneychanger.com/articles_files/book_reviews/the_mood_cure.phtml (accessed March 16, 2007).

10. Shankar Vedantam and Marc Kaufman, "Doctors Influenced by Mention of Drug Ads," *Washington Post*, April 27, 2005, A1.

11. "Depression," MayoClinic.com, http://www.mayoclinic.com/health/depression/DS00175/DSECTION=8 (accessed March 16, 2007).

12. Aaron Smith, "The Antidepressants to Watch in '06," CNNMoney.com, http://money.cnn.com/2006/01/04/news/companies/antidepressants/index.htm (accessed March 16, 2007).

13. Scott Roberts, "Generic Zoloft Approved," *HealthDay*, July 5, 2006.

14. John M. Grohol, Psy.D., "Top 20 Psychiatric Prescriptions," PsychCentral.com, http://psychcentral.com/lib/2006/08/top-20-psychiatric-prescriptions-for-2005/ (accessed August 31, 2006).

15. Michael W. Smith, M.D., ed., "Depression Recovery: An Overview," WebMD, http://www.webmd.com/depression/depression-recovery-overview (accessed November 1, 2005).

16. The Associated Press, "FDA Warns of Suicide Risk for Paxil," September 18, 2006.

17. "Depression: The Herbal Alternative," *Psychology Today*, May/June 1997, http://www.psychologytoday.com/articles/pto-19970501-000025.html (accessed March 16, 2007).

18. Balch, and Stengler, *Prescription for Natural Cures*, 185.

19. Camille Chatterjee, "Pin Down Depression," *Psychology Today*, September/October 1999, http://www.psychologytoday.com/articles/pto-19990901-000030.html (accessed March 16, 2007).

20. Dr. Jill Ammon-Wexler, "Your Second Brain," SelfGrowth.com, http://www.selfgrowth.com/articles/Wexler3.html (accessed March 16, 2007).

21. Elzy Kolb, "Serotonin: Is There Anything It Can't Do?" *The Journal of the College of Physicians and Surgeons of Columbia University* 19, no. 2 (Spring 1999).

Key #1

1. Jo Revill, "Poor Diet Link to Rising Cases of Depression" *The Observer,*, January 15, 2006, http://observer.guardian.co.uk/uk_news/story/0,6903,1686730,00.html (accessed March 16, 2007).

2. Rex Russell, *What the Bible Says About Health Living* (Ventura, CA: Regal, 1996), 62–63.

3. "What Are Essential Fatty Acids?" Barf World, http://www.barfworld.com/html/learn_more/efa.shtml (accessed March 16, 2007).

4. ABC News, "Defeating Depression: As Easy as Omega-3,"Mercola.com, http://www.mercola.com/2002/nov/30/depression.htm (accessed September 17, 2002).

5. Sally Fallon and Mary G. Enig, Ph.D., *Nourishing Traditions: The Cookbook that Challenges Politically Correct Nutrition and the Diet Dictocrats,* (Winona Lake, IN: NewTrends Publishing, 2000).

6. Diane Schwarzbein, M.D., *The Schwarzbein Principle* (Deerfield Beach, FL: Health Communications, 1999), 44.

7. Paul Schulick, *Ginger: Common Spice & Wonder Drug,* 3rd ed. (Prescott, AZ: Hohm Press, 1996), 36.

8. F. Batmanghelidj, M.D., *You're Not Sick, You're Thirsty!* (New York: Warner Books, 2003), 179.

9. Ibid, 200.

10. "Caffeine," The Stress Confidential Helpline, http://stresshelp.tripod.com/id7.html (accessed March 16, 2007).

11. *Encyclopedia of Natural Healing* (Burnaby, BC: Alive Publishing, 1997), 169.

Key #2

1. "Omega-3 Fatty Acids," University of Maryland Medical Center, http://www.umm.edu/altmed/ConsSupplements/Omega3FattyAcidscs.html (accessed March 16, 2007).

2. "Fish Oils May Benefit Manic Depression," NutriCraze, http://www.nutricraze.com/Article_about_Fish-Oils-May-Benefit-Manic-Depression-a-5547.html (accessed March 16, 2007).

3. Sid Kirchheimer, " Vitamin D May Ease Depression," WebMD, http://www.webmd.com/content/Article/91/101374.htm (accessed August 3, 2004).

4. Nancy Schimelpfening, "Vitamin for Depression?" About.com, http://depression.about.com/cs/diet/a/vitamin.htm (accessed March 16, 2007).

5. Ibid.

6. Richard P. Brown, M.D., and Patricia L. Gerbarg, M.D., *The Rhodiola Revolution* (Emmaus, PA: Rodale, 2004), 131.

7. Ibid, 132.

Key #3

1. Lisa Petrillo, "SDSU Study: Germs Hitch Ride in Plane Bathrooms," *San Diego Union-Tribune*, December 26, 2005.
2. C. J. McManus and S. T. Kelley, "Molecular Survey of Aeroplane Bacterial Contamination," *Journal of Applied Microbiology* 99, no. 3 (2005): 502–8.
3. PR Newswire Association, "Flu Season Is Here," October 6, 2005, http://www.keepmedia.com/pubs/PRNewswire/2005/10/06/1039338. (accessed June 2, 2007)

Key #4

1. Betsy McCormack, *Fit Over 40 for Dummies* (Foster City, CA: IDG Books, 2001) 54.
2. "Depression and Anxiety: Exercise Eases Symptoms," MayoClinic.com, http://www.mayoclinic.com/health/depression-and-exercise/MH00043 (accessed March 16, 2007).

Key #5

1. Mindy Pennybacker, "Healthier Home Cleaning," *The Green Guide*, September 8, 2003.

About the Authors

Jordan Rubin has dedicated his life to transforming the health of God's people one life at a time. He is the founder and chairman of Garden of Life, Inc., a health and wellness company based in West Palm Beach, Florida, that produces organic functional foods, whole food nutritional supplements, and personal care products and he's a much-in-demand speaker on various health topics.

He and his wife, Nicki, are the parents of a toddler-aged son, Joshua. They make their home in Palm Beach Gardens, Florida.

Joseph D. Brasco, MD, who has extensive knowledge and experience in gastroenterology and internal medicine, attended medical school at Medical College of Wisconsin in Milwaukee, Wisconsin, and is board certified with the American Board of Internal Medicine. Besides writing for various medical journals, he is also the coauthor of *Restoring Your Digestive Health* with Jordan Rubin. Dr. Brasco is currently in private practice in Huntsville, Alabama.

BHI

BIBLICAL HEALTH
INSTITUTE

The Biblical Health Institute (www.BiblicalHealthInstitute.com) is
an online learning community housing educational resources and
curricula reinforcing and expanding on Jordan Rubin's Biblical
Health message.

Biblical Health Institute provides:

1. **"101" level FREE**, introductory courses corresponding
   to Jordan's book The Great Physician's Rx for Health
   and Wellness and its seven keys; Current "101" courses
   include:

   * "Eating to Live 101"

   * "Whole Food Nutrition Supplements 101"

   * "Advanced Hygiene 101"

   * "Exercise and Body Therapies 101"

   * "Reducing Toxins 101"

   * "Emotional Health 101"

   * "Prayer and Purpose 101"

2. **FREE** resources (healthy recipes, what to E.A.T.,
   resource guide)

3. **FREE** media--videos and video clips of Jordan, music
   therapy samples, etc.--and much more!

Additionally, Biblical Health Institute also offers in-depth
courses for those who want to go deeper.

Course offerings include:

   * 40-hour certificate program to become a Biblical
     Health Coach

   * A la carte course offerings designed for personal study
     and growth

   * Home school courses developed by Christian
     educators, supporting home-schooled students and
     their parents (designed for middle school and high
     school ages)

**For more information and updates on these and other resources go to
www.BiblicalHealthInstitute.com**